YOU COULD BE PRIME MINISTER ONE DAY SON

– Memoir of a Baby-Boomer

DENNIS HARRISON

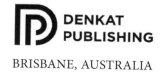

DENKAT
PUBLISHING

BRISBANE, AUSTRALIA

Website: www.denkatpublishing.com

Cover design by germancreative

Author has obtained release from copyright to use the following:

Photograph of Dennis winning the school mile at the 1963 Elwood High
School House Sports Carnival. Photograph credit Fairfax Syndication;
published in "The Age" newspaper 1963

The Second Trombonist - Photograph taken by Jocelyn Watts of Maryborough,
Queensland

Author Headshot Photograph taken by Mana Salsali of Mana Photography,
Brisbane.

Article written by Ian Howarth and published in "Australian Financial Review
on June 19th, 1991 entitled "Crusader wins Court Dispute with Santos" Release
granted by Ian Howarth.

To my father, written in your honour,
I am forever grateful.
And to families everywhere,
the cornerstone of our society.

AUTHOR'S NOTE

Real names are used for:

- Harrison family members, Mum (Hazel), Dad (Milton), brother Brian, Pa and Ma Harrison, Joy (Aunt Joy), Kathy, my wife, and our children Nicole (Nicki), Suzanne (Suzie), Therese (Tess), and our grandchildren, Catherine, Patrick and Thomas

- Martin family members, Edmund (Uncle Ted) Martin, Aunty Eve, Neville (Nev), and Graeme.

- Ron Richards (Uncle Ron).

- Mr. Will, my Elwood High School Maths teacher.

- Miss Rowan, Elwood High School Senior mistress.

- Elwood High School students Sonya Varga and Robert de Klyne.

- Political, entertainment, religious, and sporting identities.

- Some industry and geological identities.

It was very important to honour the careers of Edmund (Ted) Martin and Ron Richards. I was able to establish the details of Ted's cricketing career from the magnificent Trove database. Ron Richards' career in the Australian Security Intelligence Organisation (ASIO) is a matter of public record as documented in "The Spy Catchers–The Original History of ASIO 1949-1963" by David Horner.

All other names are fictitious, but of course based on real people in my life. I have been faithful to my memory, but others may remember things differently. The work contains interpretations of events that may be solely mine. The interactions described within are in many cases fancifully elaborated and enhanced to advance the story. For me the story is the driver, told to illuminate understanding and entertain. There is no intent to humiliate or embarrass anyone. If indeed I have erred in this, I unreservedly apologise. I chose to use fictitious names for most other people in the memoir to preserve their anonymity. Sometimes a character may be a composite of many characters.

Contents

Author's Note.. v

Prologue xi

Part 1 - Childhood 1946 – 1960 13

  1   Roots Of Pugilism 15

  2   Uncertain Start 17

  3   Near Miss Incident 19

  4   Scrapings Off The Vats 23

  5   Daisy Nielsen 25

  6   Early Delusions Of Power...................................... 27

  7   Under The Pump Think Creatively 29

  8   Mucking Around With Robbie 33

  9   Organised Pugilism... 37

10   A Serious Incident... 39

11   Life Around The Water 41

12   Give Me That Old Time Religion 47

13   The Danger Of Three Seater Lounges 51

14   Life After Death.. 57

15   Cricket Lessons... 59

16   The Art Of Cricket By Edmund Martin................ 63

17   Mental Illness.. 69

18   Thwarted Musical Ambitions 73

19   Fifteen Is A Good Average 77

20 Chasing Daisy Nielsen Ends Badly 81

21 Perth Modern School 85

22 Maybe Billy Graham Can Help 89

Part 2 - Adolescence 1960 – 1968 93

23 Clickety Clack 95

24 How He Grow Up So Big Then? 99

25 More Than A Project 103

26 The Letter 107

27 Let's Start Again 111

28 I Hear You Mastered Huntingdale 117

29 Equal Dux Form Three 121

30 Inspired By Mr Will 125

31 The Richmond Methodists 129

32 Drama At The Palais Theatre 135

33 School Mile Triumph 141

34 My Adolescent Mates 143

35 A Wee Bit Of Road Rage 147

36 Excursions Into Science 149

37 White Boots 151

38 Surrounded By Purple 155

39 Almost All Over Red Rover 161

40 Becoming A Geologist 167

41 Lucky Rabbit Lucky Dennis 173

42 Another Near Miss 179

43 The Fanta Must Have Been Off 183

44   Oh No A Purple Sports Coat 191

45   Down The Platform I Looked 195

Part 3 - Adulthood 1968 – 1991 .... **205**

46   Dennis Harrison, Who? 207

47   Dr Geert Van Der Welle 211

48   On Assignment In Wewak, New Guinea 215

49   Snake! Snake! Snake! 221

50   Looking Into The Abyss Again 225

51   Mutiny On The Sepik 231

52   Under Duress Science Of No Help 235

53   The Panhandle Sets In The West 237

54   Trees Don't Talk Back 239

55   Yours Truly Shuts Down Nt Railways 245

56   Career Moves 255

57   The Caravan Story 259

58   Uncle Ted's Lessons Finally Pay Off 265

59   More Career Moves 269

60   Meteoric Rise And Rapid Fall 275

61   He Gave Us Our Values You Know 281

62   A Dash At Politics 285

63   David Over Goliath Victory 289

Part 4 - Maturity 1991 – 2016 .... **295**

64   It Can All Change In A Moment 297

65   I Knew I Had Lost My Best Mate 301

66   Mid Life Crisis 305

67   Big Jo Jo Hohepa 311

68   Like Fine Wine A Geologist Matures............315

69   Oh, I Play Second Trombone 319

Epilogue.. **325**

Acknowledgements................................ **331**

About The Author................................ **332**

PROLOGUE

I am a post-war baby boomer. I was born on the 6th of August, 1946, which happened to be the first anniversary of the atomic bomb dropping on Hiroshima. Born a Leo, I have an affinity for big cats and the lion.

When I was only about four years old, my mother knitted a red jumper with a magnificent lion on the front. The lion, standing on his hind legs, had raised front legs with claws extended. It felt appropriate. I felt powerful.

In 1998, when my wife Kathy & I were taking our first overseas trip to Switzerland, we saw the Lion of Lucerne. It measures at a staggering 10 meters in length, six meters in height and it was carved into the cliff face of a quarry. Back then I wrote:

"The pain, the loyalty, the passion, the service ...... the most expressive piece of sculpture in Europe." And I still feel it that deeply when I look at this photo today. This reverberates in my bones, in my soul. The lion fought and served without question until the very end. Notice the broken tip of a spear in his flank. It was the final battle that had caused his death, but not before he had fought and broken the shaft of the spear at the tip. The expression on his face, "Well, what else would you do with your life but fight to the end defending the king, queen, country and your family?"

The growth to maturity is encapsulated in the gaining of courage. Much of my courage came from my father by his example of fortitude through adversity. His faith and belief in me has been a cornerstone to my existence. He would often tell me, "You could be prime minister one day, son."

Of course, we are made and formed by many. Male mentors are so essential for the development of a boy and, in addition to my father, I was so fortunate to have had Uncle Ted, Robbie Flood, Mr Will, Ron Richards, and Dave Slipper. Through them, I discovered the lion within.

My mother gave me religion and music, both of which I find pivotal to my existence and a great comfort. She also gave me insecurity, an insecurity that has haunted me for much of my life.

Both of my parents gave me a love of books and a thirst for knowledge. I write so that I may understand. I write with gratitude to my parents, I honour them. I respect their sacrifices.

I write with thanks to my wife and soul mate Kathy. Together over fifty years, we have celebrated so much together. You have given me tremendous support and the freedom to grow.

To our three children, we have given our best.

To our three grandchildren, may this book assist you in unravelling the great mystery of life. Any one of you could be prime minister one day!

This is my story.

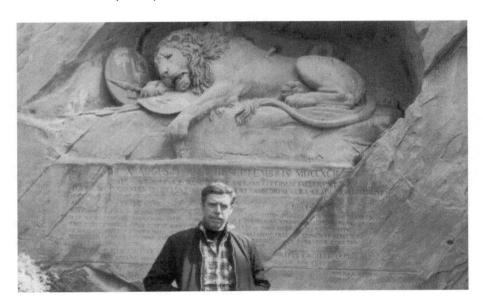

PART 1 - CHILDHOOD 1946 – 1960

"How do we get to know a person?
Through stories. All the wild and sad and courageous tales that we tell — they are what reveal us to others."

John Eldredge

1

ROOTS OF PUGILISM

I was quite manic. He had caught me early on in the fight with a right hook, but I was not backing down. Blood poured from my nose. I wiped it on my forearm and snorted it up until I nearly gagged. When that didn't work, I said to myself 'stuff that' and spread as much blood as I could across my face. I needed to go beyond the anger that was festering in my heart. I was going to get even by fair means or foul. Older by six months, and heavier, he was tough as nails, but I was quicker and mentally agile. We stood apart and circled, each wary of the next move.

I gave a few short jabs that caught his cheek. I forced myself not to speak. The fighter with the greatest fear speaks first. Watch his eyes and watch his fists, but make sure to look into his eyes. Stare him down. All this chatter was going on in my mind as we continued to circle. Light on your feet, up on your toes, don't get caught flat-footed. Where did this self-knowledge come from? After all, I was only seven years old. He and I were best mates but we fought regularly. Physical sparring, threats and dares, these were all parts of growing up, and it was inexplicably primal. The continual confrontation, measuring up and testing was the surefire way to manhood.

Robbie broke the silence. 'You are off your brain, just like your mother.'

'You prick. Don't talk about my mother like that!'

That's how the fight had started anyways. His words increased my inner resolve and I broke through his defences to land a punch square on his nose, soon following with another that split his lip.

It was then I spotted Mrs Flood heading towards us from the front door of her house.

I backed away from Robbie saying, 'Don't you ever say that about my mother again.' I turned on my heels and bolted home. When I got there, I tried to creep around the back, only to be met by my father who was gardening. He stated the obvious.

'You been fighting again, Dennis?'

'Yeah,' I replied, putting on a look of remorse because the last thing I wanted was follow-up punishment from my father.

'What was it about?'

'Robbie was saying things about Mum.'

'What sort of things?'

'That she was crazy and that everyone on the street knows.'

I saw him swallow hard and fight back his own emotions.

'Come here, son. Let's clean you up before Mum sees you,' Dad said.

We walked together into the old wooden laundry room which stood separate from the house. He gently dabbed my face with a flannel and then tended to my bloodied knuckles. Tears formed in his eyes and rolled down his cheek.

'What's Robbie look like?' he asked.

'Much worse than me.'

'Well done, son. You stood up for the family, but don't make a habit of this. It can get you into lots of trouble.'

He drew me in and gave me a hug. With a hot breath, he spoke into my ear, 'Tell Mum you fell off your bike.'

We became very close after that. A bond had formed telling me that together, we could overcome anything. I knew he was in my corner and I was certainly in his.

2

UNCERTAIN START

I was born into darkness in a mental asylum. It was going to take me a long time to see the light. There was so much confusion. The fear generated by a lack of security needed to be processed. I latched onto anything that was extended to me in love.

They hadn't actually lied to me. I had been told I was born in Subiaco, but I had immediately jumped to the conclusion that I was born in St John of God's Hospital like so many other Western Australians. I was in my fifties before I discovered that I was born at the Kensington Nursing Home in Heytesbury Road, Subiaco. My mother was in and out of mental institutions, suffering from breakdowns that I never really understood. When this happened, I would be whisked away to my grandparents' house or to my aunts and uncles. I gathered that there was some sort of shame involved with this, but it was always beyond my comprehension. I only had one older brother, Brian, and he was seven years older than me. It was too big an age gap for us to be close and having a dysfunctional family didn't help. As the youngest, they told me as little as possible and shielded me from the worst.

Back in the mid-twentieth century, nobody really knew anything about mental illness. When she was feeling up, Mum would be the life of the party. She had boundless energy and was extraordinarily capable. She could be the grand entertainer with a beautiful singing voice as well as a talented piano player. She even produced some amazing paintings in her early life. And her sponge cakes were simply the best. One of the measuring sticks of a women's domestic prowess back then was the quality of their sponge cakes, and hers were always the lightest and the fluffiest. Full female domesticity at the time demanded a capability for making clothes. She was extraordinarily gifted in this area with her needlework, knitting, crocheting and embroidery.

She had all these gifts, but the cycle would eventually turn as it had always done and we would all see irrationality creep into her daily life. Verbal jousts would become more intense between Mum and Dad, and that was when Brian and I would make ourselves scarce. There would be screaming and tears. If it got too bad, well it was off to grandma's house again. There would be no explanations, just "Oh, Mum's not well again." We were supposed to make sense of that.

She was never diagnosed with bipolar disorder. They didn't have a term for this illness back then, let alone the right drugs to manage it. What a different life she would have had now that the illness is manageable. I slowly realised that there were times that Mum just couldn't cope, and as a result I learned to walk on eggshells. Don't rock the boat. Take care of what you say and do. Assist always. Be circumspect. Artificial happiness was the safest way to adapt and survive.

It was the uncertainty, however, that was the worst. What sort of household would it be tonight? Would it be sweet peas and roses, or would I be going home to a thunderstorm or unfathomable sadness? The illness left its mark on each of us in different ways, but we were family.

3

NEAR MISS INCIDENT

My Mum, Hazel, lived in a haze most of the time. It seemed like she would lose something after each breakdown. The loss of trust and respect was cumulative. The re-building of character and life was immensely challenging. She undoubtedly loved me, and I returned that love as best I could but there was a kind of overbearing smothering that went on. She expressed fear during her depression and pleaded for forgiveness in her mania. Making sense of the inconsistency was much more than what an immature developing mind could handle. What solace can a young child give a parent that is in tears, wringing their hands whilst seated under a tree in the backyard still dressed in her nightie at three in the afternoon when coming home from school?

'What's wrong Mum?' I asked. Drawing me tight to her bosom she responded, 'I don't know. I am just sad love.'

Brian would not be home for an hour and a half and Dad for at least three hours. I needed to survive. I needed to have a strategy.

'Come inside and let's sing a happy song,' I told her.

I took her hand and we walked inside to the piano.

'What would you like to hear?'

'I'd like I've Got A Pocketful of Dreams Mum.' And she would start to play, a little hesitantly at first but then more determined. She knew her repertoire of pieces so well that she could play them all without reading the music. Even to this day I am amazed by that level of skill. So, she instinctively played on. When she dropped into reflective, moody numbers I would try to drag her back into happier ones.

'How about Happy Days Are Here Again Mum?' I asked. It lifted my mood, but not my mother's because she turned to me with tears streaming down her cheeks. She followed that up just for my benefit with You Must Have Been a Beautiful Baby.

'I'll be alright now, Dennis. Why don't you go outside and play?'

'Okay, thanks Mum.' I snuck out the back door to go find Robbie. Surely, I could find an excuse to have another fight with him just to ease the pain.

****

It was not all downtime though. Her manic ups were highly productive. I owe my love of books and music to my mother. She taught me to love books by reading them to me regularly. She prepared me well for school. I was scoring nine out of ten in Infants for reading, and the remarks on the report card said, Dennis is very sound in all his work and has an excellent general knowledge. The report cards from year to year ranged from very good to quite poor, driven no doubt by the ups and downs of family harmony as well as the inherent anger and confusion that bounced around within me.

I learned early on in life to enjoy my own company. It was a natural outcome given the fact that I was with a brother seven years my senior with his own life and emotions to sort out, a mother with extended periods of either being mentally lost or physically absent, and a father who had to keep it all together as best he could by developing a career and maintaining a stable income. This isolation drove me into a world of books. The books allowed an escape from reality and a means of making sense of, and interpreting, life.

To her credit, whatever musical ability and interest I now have is something that I owe to my mother. I was assigned to a strict German piano teacher named Mrs Schmidt for three years. She advanced me to grade three until my music ceased during one of her episodes. But while Mum was up, she was strong enough to control me after school insisting that I practice for a half an hour before I could go outside and play with Robbie and any of my other mates. She also knew if I was faking practice or not concentrating. 'That's not right, Dennis,' she would call out from the kitchen, and if it was complete rubbish she would appear and, after wiping her hands on her apron, would demonstrate how it was done. 'That's the way it should go, Dennis. Now you have a go, and when you get it right you can go outside.' It was tough discipline for a young lad who just wanted to get out and play cricket or kick a football.

Getting to Mrs Schmidt was not that easy. I had to walk two blocks and catch a trolley-bus to Wembley from our house in Floreat Park. This presented interesting challenges for a young child. My parents had presented me with a small brown Globite case to carry my music. I suppose I should say that I was proud of it, but this music caper was just something I did to keep peace in the household. I was expected to cooperate.

I had little concept of time and minimal organisational ability, which meant that I was forever running to catch the bus. On one of my wild exits from the house and sprints through bushland, I felt this sharp pain in my foot. A palm needle had penetrated itself deeply into my foot just beneath my big toe. I dropped the music case and fell to the ground screaming in pain. I was very fortunate because Mrs Flood saw the accident and came running to my aid. She extracted the needle with a few yelps from me, but I bravely held back any tears because Robbie was watching. Mrs Flood sent me on my way with a dab of Dettol and a bandaged foot. I limped to the bus stop and caught a later bus.

I should not be here to tell this tale as on another occasion, going to Mrs Schmidt's, there was a more serious incident than the palm needle. I had entered a dream state of complete relaxation when I looked out of the trolley-bus window only to see that it had passed the stop that I had to get off at. Without another thought, I grabbed my music case and jumped off the bus which was now moving at great speed. I hit the bitumen at a pace that made it impossible to stay upright, and I came to rest in the gutter having managed to roll over like a ball. By some sort of divine providence, there were no cars trailing the trolley-bus or attempting to pass on the inside or else I would have been killed.

I managed to stand up and everything seemed to move okay, no broken bones. Deep scratches had been carved into my music case. Oh hell, I thought. I'll have to tell my parents a story about how this beautiful case was now in a state of disrepair. I walked back to Mrs Schmidt's house, climbed the stairs, and sat on the chair outside her music room. Daisy Nielsen came out of the room. She was a schoolmate of mine and I had a crush on her. She had attractive blonde curls that bounced around as she walked, and sweet moist lips. On this day, however, I left my eyes downcast and didn't even greet her. Mrs Schmidt yelled, 'Your turn, Dennis.' I picked up my case and limped into the room. She had one look at me and exclaimed, 'Vat has happened vith you, Dennis?'

'I have had a bit of an accident, Mrs Schmidt.'

'Look at you. Let me clean you up, you poor boy.'

I then discovered that Mrs Schmidt had her own bottle of Dettol. When she had finished patching me up she said, 'No lesson today. How about a cup of hot cocoa and some pikelets?'

4

SCRAPINGS OFF THE VATS

Robbie and I were a couple of street urchins. We never had any money, so somehow we just got by with our smarts. We would ride down to the corner of Birkdale Street and Cambridge Street and hang around Mr Phillips' fish and chips shop.

'You got any scrapings Mr Phillips?' I asked.

'Hang around for a minute. Just need a couple more paying customers,' he'd reply.

And sure enough, after two more customers came and went he called us in.

'There you go boys, make it last.'

Mr Phillips would thrust into our hands a piece of white paper soaked in oil with a skerrick of scrapings from the surface of his vats. Sometimes he would even throw in a couple of chips.

'Now skedaddle. You're not good for my business hanging around like you do. We're not a charity you know.'

Mr Phillips was more than generous with us so I went back to his shop years later and bought some fish and chips. The business was then run by his son. I knew it was his son because he had the same large, curved, and hawkish nose as his father. Well out of earshot of Mr Phillips, we used to talk about his big nose. 'You could hide an unshelled peanut up his nose, you could,' Robbie would remark. 'No you couldn't. It wouldn't get around the corner,' I would respond. We invented bigger and better stories each time until we broke down in laughter.

5

DAISY NIELSEN

Robbie and I grew up in the era of 'be seen but not heard,' and we did just about everything together. The young suburb of Floreat Park in the early 1950s was a patchwork quilt of houses separated from each other with undeveloped bush blocks. We had a half mile walk to school along a fairly flat road with the final leg of it through bushland. Whether we walked together or not depended upon the latest state of play of our combative friendship. Oftentimes, I would take the walk by myself so I guess Robbie and I must have ended most days with a tiff.

I would attack the walk to school as a slow ramble because there were always distractions along the way, the vacant blocks hiding bird nests, goannas, and lizards. I cannot recall ever being in trouble for arriving late to school. Mum must have dispatched me with plenty of time to spare. She would send me off with my little leather bag strapped over my shoulders. The bag held very little, just some pencils, an exercise book, a reader, and of course my lunch. Lunch was a simple affair of two sandwiches, cheese and vegemite were my favourite, but it could be as simple as jam or honey and a piece of fruit. The fruit was not always consumed. I still remember the foul stench of a fetid banana that had been left in the bag for weeks. The black mess had permanently impregnated the leather at the bottom of the bag. To this day, I have an inability to eat bananas with black skin because of this childhood experience.

Another good aspect of the walk to school was that it took me past Daisy Nielsen's house. Her house was backed onto parkland that had several large gum trees, and she had a cubby house on the back fence alongside the park. One day while walking home after school,

I got bold and approached the fence line. I could hear Daisy playing in her cubby house and I spoke to her through the fence.

'Is that you, Daisy?'

'Yes. Who is that?'

'Dennis.'

'Dennis who?'

'Dennis Harrison. How many Dennises do you know?'

'Oh, Dennis.'

'Are you alone in there?'

'Yes.'

'Can I come and play with you?' I asked.

'Sure, but how are you going to get over the fence.'

'I'll find a way.'

I dragged some branches over to the fence and created a makeshift staircase, and before you could say Jack Robinson I was over the fence and inside Daisy's cubby house. It took my eyes some time to adjust as it was quite dark in there.

'Let's play doctors and nurses,' she said. It all started quite innocently until she said, 'I'll show you mine if you show me yours.'

'How do you play that?' I asked.

'Well you know we are a bit different down there. You show me your willy and I show you my milly. You go first,' she said. This was all very new to me and right when I had my pants down around my ankles, I heard Mrs Nielsen approaching the cubby house.

'I've got some lemonade and biscuits for you, Daisy.'

I was out of there in a flash and managed to scale the fence before Mrs Nielsen opened the cubby house door. My sexual education would have to wait for another day.

6

EARLY DELUSIONS OF POWER

I was born on the first anniversary of the bombing of Hiroshima. I often wonder if that was another metaphysical reason I was prone to violence and conflict. However, observing the continual trauma and tension between my parents was the more likely cause. The lesson I took from those turbulent years was to fight and survive, the Darwinian instinct of survival. I remember being disruptive even in kindergarten. I advanced to first year primary school, and during the big lunchtime breaks I concocted a game where I corralled as many girls as I could into a bark humpy. I then had to patrol the borders of the humpy to protect my girls from other threatening, roaming boys. These were my girls and not to be shared. It was like I had my own harem. Of course, Daisy would be the first I would attract into the humpy. How I managed to do this is beyond my memory or even my current imagination. Could have been my jam or honey sandwiches I suppose, but my ego says it must have been my natural charm. Alas, I had skills in my youth that never advanced into adulthood.

To enter the classroom we used to have to line up in two rows, boys in one row and girls alongside in the other. I worked out that it was good to stay towards the back of the row, and when the teachers were not looking I could just lean over and give one of the girls a kiss. I made sure they were in my harem and not just any girl. It was a lot of fun until, in a fit of jealousy, Daisy announced to one of the teachers at the top of her voice, 'Miss Roberts! Dennis Harrison just kissed Janice Stephens!'

Miss Roberts came bustling down the line. She brushed past the blushing Janice and pulled me aside.

'Did you kiss Janice, Dennis?'

'I think I might have Miss Roberts.'

'You can't do that. Just stand in line and leave the girls alone.'

'Yes Miss. It's so very hard though Miss. I like girls, they are so beautiful.'

'Enough of that Dennis or you'll go to see the headmaster.'

'Yes Miss.'

7

UNDER THE PUMP THINK CREATIVELY

I was destined to have several visits with the headmaster. I don't believe that I was inherently bad, I was just a spirited tearaway kid that didn't know any better. On opening day in *Infants* I won the fifty-metre sprint. I thought that was pretty good but Dad behaved as though I had won a gold medal in the Olympics. He was so proud and gushing. What made it even better for him was that his father, my Pa Harrison, was there also. I think Mum was there too but I can't remember. She could have been having one of her turns, or Dad just took over and dominated and didn't leave any space for her.

Winning the race set a pattern that was to continue for most of my life - never let the old man down and behave in ways that would make him proud. He was always so supportive and encouraging. Encouragement enables, discouragement disables, and a catch phrase he used in my adolescence, and adult life, that he loved to repeat was, 'You could be prime minister one day, son.' What a guy to have in your corner, and this was all done regardless of his own immense suffering.

I probably suffered from small person syndrome. In my experience, it's mostly the short people that are the fastest to rise to the bait. Taller people are slower to both react and cause trouble. Mind you there are exceptions to that rule. I remember there was a large, overweight boy named Michael Henderson who liked to throw his weight around. We ended up in a fight down on the sports field. We were surrounded by a pack of kids yelling, 'Fight, fight, fight!' And for the life of me, I can't remember what we were even fighting about. Somehow, I had overcome him and I was sitting on top of his soft midriff pounding him with punches. I had beaten him into submission. 'Stop, stop,' he pleaded. 'Stop, I get migraines.' At the time, I hadn't yet developed compassion or a large vocabulary. I stopped only for a brief moment saying, 'Better your brains than my brains.' Then I continued swinging blow after blow. There are no knock out blows when it comes to childish punches so fights can go on interminably. The commotion did eventually attract a teacher though. I was dragged off him and without negotiation frogmarched to the headmaster for a caning.

Primary school seemed like a time of boundless energy and exploration. I was always testing the limits of what you could and could not get away with. There was a radio show back then called 'Yes What?' that was very popular, and it was set in a classroom involving the interaction of a teacher with his pupils Greenbottle, Bottomley, and Stamford amongst others. The show would commence with the ringing of the school bell. The pupils were extremely disrespectful of the dithering teacher that could not keep control over them. They were forever playing pranks and telling creative lies about all and sundry, distracting the teacher away from the teaching roll. It was very funny and the quick wit, double entendre, and innuendo expanded my vocabulary and understanding of life. I can now see it was a great way to learn many things, but the downside was the complete lack of respect, fairness, and bullying nature of the children's behaviour upon the poor teacher who could not cope with it. I was to see this repeated in my secondary schooling days as well.

Today, a show like this would be banned. There would be a public outcry by educationalists. In addition to the humour, the show provided many learning experiences, however it was the antithesis of cooperation. It set up a win-lose equation and the teacher was forever losing. A young brain cannot differentiate between acceptable and unacceptable behaviour after all. In one of the episodes, Greenbottle filled up a water pistol with ink from the ink well and squirted Bottomley and Stamford with it. He ended up being sent to the headmaster's office for the behaviour. What prompted me to emulate this behaviour? It provoked the same response. Off to the headmaster's office.

It was a long walk to the headmaster's office and I was not escorted there by the teacher. Left to my own devices, I dragged my feet very slowly, trying to work out how you sensibly explain why you would fill a water pistol with ink and fire it around the classroom, fully knowing this was one of my more monumental stuff-ups. The walk took me past the cloakroom where all the raincoats were hung. It was winter in Perth and there were wet raincoats hanging on all the pegs. Inspiration came to me like a flash from heaven. I could escape punishment. I walked into the cloakroom and sat down to carefully plan out my next moves. I allowed about fifteen minutes to lapse in order to incorporate the walk to and from the office, and I then selected a suitable wet coat and rubbed my hands up and down on one of the sleeves until they were red and raw. I walked back to the classroom in the rain which made it easier to turn on the mock tears. I entered the classroom with two red hands prominently displayed, hamming up the mock tears and legs shaking. The leg shaking was real because by now I was having doubts about my ability to get away with this charade. I walked to my desk and sat down.

'Let that be a lesson to you, Dennis.'

'Yes Miss Roberts,' I responded head down. 'It won't happen again.'

I got away with my charade and I had learned another valuable life lesson. When under the pump, think creatively. Real wisdom would, however, be somewhat delayed.

8

MUCKING AROUND WITH ROBBIE

The competition between Robbie and me was relentless. It was both while at school and after school. We were both good at sports. In our final year at the school, he was captain of the football team and vice-captain of the cricket team. I was captain of the cricket team and vice-captain of the football team. I had a big edge on the cricket front because I had Uncle Ted. Uncle Ted had been a first-class cricketer and I learned everything from him.

Robbie and I would organise knock-up games of football and cricket in the park at the bottom of our hill. We were always opposing captains. It helped that we supplied the balls, bats, and stumps. We would select our sides from the collection of young specimens in the park and those that we had dragged from the adjacent backyards. We were always the keenest and best players. It was all about us and our contest. The others were there to make up the numbers. We would play until dark.

Mr Flood was a plumber. He drove around in a battered old van with "Flood Plumbing" painted on its side, along with the phrase, 'Got a flood? Call a Flood to fix it.' He had turned an unfortunate surname in his line of business into an asset. He had four sons, all conveniently spaced about four years apart. You would think that Mr Flood had designed it that way as a part of his business plan. Each of his boys would only complete the compulsory minimum schooling and then be ensconced as the latest recruit to the business. Robbie was the youngest Flood and still had some fun years ahead before life would catch up to him and become all serious.

As the youngest son, Robbie grew up tough just to survive. I admired his courage. Robbie could somehow always climb to a higher branch on the big pine trees out in the front of our houses. I had never seen him cry, and Robbie had had some bad accidents. He fell out of the pine tree once and broke his arm. I had fetched Mrs Flood and despite his twisted arm with a bone sticking out through his wound, he didn't even whimper. I was telling Mum and Dad about it that night over dinner. 'He didn't cry but he was very white and not saying much. I think he hit his head on the ground as well.' It was the wrong thing to have done, bringing up Robbie's unfortunate accident at the dinner table, because I just got admonished by Mum yet again to not go climbing on those pine trees. Mum was always a drag on my courage; she was so protective.

I developed a love of books early in life. Again, I have to thank Mum for that. I used to listen to Biggles and Hop Harrigan on the radio, and of course Greenbottle. I would read Enid Blyton's Famous Five, Robinson Crusoe, and all sorts of coloured religious books that Mum kept throwing my way. I vividly remember the cover of two books but do not know their titles. One was predominantly green with a deer and its fawn with their beautiful speckled coats. I cannot remember much of the story but I was taken by the beauty of the creatures, their exposure to danger, and the alertness and speed required for their very survival. They were sensitive and beautiful, and they were hunted. The other book had a black panther on the cover. The panther was crouching on a rock making itself as small and as invisible as possible, slinking forward ever so slowly with its wide yellow eyes, about to pounce upon its prey. It represented the hunter. It was dangerous, powerful, in control of its own destiny, and maybe even sinister, although I didn't think about that aspect at the time.

I must have been attracted more to the panther as I formed 'The Black Panther Club.' I made up membership cards. Robbie and I were the only members and we would play games in the bush block two houses down from us. We would solve crimes like Larry Kent, a suave radio show detective, and win army battles.

It was about then when Robbie had a big accident. While riding our bikes past the local park we had spotted a bird's nest high up in a tree. This certainly needed to be examined. It was interesting enough, but unfortunately there were no eggs. We returned to our bikes. Robbie had flung his down over a drainage grate and as he went to pick it up he noticed some silver coins at the bottom of the drain. We managed to lift the heavy grate before Robbie jumped down and recovered the coins. He no sooner had said, 'We've got enough for some real fish and chips now,' when the grate dropped down into place chopping his big toe off. We both peered into the grate until he passed out.

I had another bonzer dinner time story for Mum and Dad that night. 'I ran for Mrs Flood because Robbie passed out. You should have seen it. There was blood everywhere. But Robbie didn't cry at all, you know.'

That accident was a great leveller in our competitive battle for male dominance. Now I could climb the pine tree a lot higher. Before the accident, we were evenly matched at football but now I was faster, and I knew just when to bump Robbie to make him go off the ball.

9

ORGANISED PUGILISM

Sometime after the toe-cutting incident whilst we were in the bush shack on 'Black Panther' business, Robbie pissed on my leg. He claimed it was an accident, but I took offence.

'What's wrong with you! Can't you piss straight?'

'Me Mum stuck a safety pin through me donga when I was in nappies. It comes out the side sometimes. Makes a 'Flood' everywhere,' he laughed.

'Does not. You did that on purpose.'

'Did not. I lost my balance because of me lost big toe.'

'You're having me on, ya liar!'

'Am not. Cross me heart and hope to choke.'

'Like hell.'

'What ya gonna do about it?'

'I'm gonna have ya, that's what,' I snapped.

And then it was on. We were at it, throwing punches and wrestling each other to the ground. There was so much commotion that both of our older brothers, Brian and Gary, came to the rescue and pulled us apart. They sent us off our separate ways. I remembered getting home and peering out from behind the lounge room curtains. Brian and Gary were in deep conversation for some time. Then they shook hands and parted. I dropped the curtain and made myself scarce in the backyard.

The big fight had occurred only a fortnight before Christmas. I got a great surprise on Christmas Day. Brian had bought me some boxing gloves as a gift.

'Wow! Thanks, Brian. Can't wait to show Robbie.'

'He'll have a pair as well,' Brian said.

'How do you know?'

'Gary and I made a deal. You two are going to fight properly now. If you and Robbie want a fight, you can do it with Gary and me present and with these gloves on.'

Our fights were now done with a sense of sportsmanship under the supervision of Brian and Gary. They would mark out a make shift square with some white paint underneath the big pine tree. They would hold their protégés back and then say, '*Go get him!*' as though we were a couple of dogs. We would race together and belt into each other. The two older boys would pull us apart at regular intervals so that we could cool down. They would give us some words of wisdom and then we would be off into it again. I remember seeing Brian and Gary winking at each other. They were getting a great return on their investment.

10
A SERIOUS INCIDENT

Robbie nearly killed me once. We were riding down to the shops to get a refund for returning all the soft drink bottles. I had a string bag full of the bottles over the handle bars. Now, Robbie had a lot of adjusting to do after he lost his big toe to the grate. His balance was real crooked there for a while. He had just swerved his bike into mine and I fell off and landed on all those broken bottles. I had a piece of glass stuck in the soft part of my wrist below my hand. There was blood everywhere. I ran home up the hill with blood spurting out of my wrist about nine inches high on every heartbeat. I had cut one and half tendons and an artery.

I made it up the front stairs to the front door of the house and collapsed. Mum went into a panic and rang for an ambulance, and then she rang Dad. She told them both that I had been hit by a car. Brian responded very well, placing a towel over my wrist and elevating it on a chair. Dad arrived home before the ambulance despite having a longer distance to drive. I was taken off to the Royal Children's Hospital in Subiaco under police escort. It impressed Robbie and that was important to me. It was one of the highlights of my life to that point and gave me great prestige with Robbie.

The doctor gave me a mask and told me to breathe in deeply after him on the count, one, two, three... I was down for the count under chloroform.

11

LIFE AROUND THE WATER

We did lots of things with the Martins. Aunty Eve was Uncle Ted's wife and Mum's sister. They had two sons, Nev and Graeme, who were just like Brian and me, seven years apart but each one year older than us. We had lots of holidays together on Rottnest Island and in Mandurah. Nev and Brian would pair off and do their own thing while Graham and I would play together. The adults would enjoy each other's company on the beach, picnicking, fishing, and playing bridge together until all hours of the night.

Mum and Aunty Eve were a couple of good looking women, looking great in their one-piece bathing outfits; bikinis had not been around at that time. We had many Easter holidays on Rottnest Island. No vehicles were allowed on the island, only bikes. Each morning we would all ride out and check the two crayfish pots. It was hard for Graeme and me to keep up with the adults with our small-wheeled bikes. Mum and Aunty Eve would sleep in. It was exciting arriving home and emptying the hessian bags on the kitchen floor to watch the crayfish scramble around.

Graeme and I had the task to ride down to the bakery and buy the hot cross buns. There was nothing better than to have a hot cross bun straight from the oven with a thick spread of butter and raspberry jam. One Easter we had a cottage and in the cabin alongside there were two hot single ladies. They would sunbake out on their lilos, all oiled up for tanning in their swim suits. Graeme and I would creep up behind the bushes that separated the two cottage yards and perve and fantasise. I named my girl Rosemary Clooney, and Graeme's girl was Rita Hayworth. By going to the pictures, we had learned from our dads that Rosemary and Rita were something to look at. To our inexperienced eyes, they were a couple of stunners. Our parents would play cards to all hours of the night and we would be put in the same bed with our heads at opposite ends. We used to try and outdo each other by taking it in turns to tell imaginative stories. Graeme's stories always seemed more involved and interesting than mine. Larry Kent and Biggles' stories were the best, but that Easter we created a lot of Rosemary and Rita stories.

****

All our fishing with the Martins up until that point was with hand lines off the beach and the rocks, until the summer Dad decided to make a boat. Dad was good with his hands. He worked briefly as a furniture salesman and admired the art of French polishing. He had a great eye for shape and form and good craftsmanship. I learned from him that utility was good but there was a beauty to be found beyond the sheer usefulness of objects. What I didn't learn from him, however, was how to be useful with my hands. He was an impatient man and a rotten teacher. He insisted on doing it all himself with no idea of team work or delegating tasks. Nothing was done calmly; there was always a sense of urgency and drama as though the whole project was on the edge of failure. He had a big barrel chest built up as a young man due to rowing in eights on the Swan River.

The boat was to be constructed under cover on the back veranda that had been added to the initial house. This was my Dad's, Milton's, first boat, although prior to this he had made a Canadian canoe. He had completed secondary school and beyond that had self-educated. He was an inquisitive man that had a thirst for knowledge and read widely. He liked to know how things worked so he would read practical magazines on cars, woodworking, and 'how to' manuals. He was a good and proud gardener and worked his butt off to keep the house in order.

He was a proud man and his barrel chest looked even bigger on the day he declared the boat finished. There was only one problem: he had got the dimensions of the boat and the exit door from the veranda all wrong. The boat was landlocked and couldn't fit through the veranda door. We kids became scarce because there was more cursing than usual, and would you want to be around when your father has egg on his face? Even Mum was alert enough to be careful with her words that day.

The resourceful man overcame the problem by dismantling the louvered windows, pulling some trees out of the garden, and the boat was man-hauled over the wall and out into the backyard. We all slept easier once that project was over.

****

The boat transformed our holidays with the Martins. We started going to Mandurah for Easter and the long Christmas holidays. Mandurah is the second-largest city in Western Australia, located approximately 72 kilometres south of the capital, Perth. It is a fabulous place for swimming and fishing. A five-kilometre channel passes through the town and runs into the ocean. Upstream from the channel is the massive Harvey estuary, fed by the Harvey, Serpentine, and Murray Rivers. At the northern part of the Harvey Inlet is the large, shallow Peel Inlet. It is a breeding ground for blue swimmer crabs.

Crabbing provided us with great sport. The adults would stay on the boat and let it drift with the wind across the shallow beds of estuary sand, weed, and mud. We four boys would be thrown overboard with a homemade crab scoop net, made from fencing wire mounted on the end of a broomstick. The estuary had a thin layer of white sand that sat on top of a dark blue-black mud. The crabs would mate, spawn, and rest up in little blue mud hollows, and the technique was to prod the hole with the bare end of the broomstick. If there was a crab in the hole, it would come out all mad with its claws extended and move from side to side. Once caught in the net, we would walk back to the boat and one of the adults would measure the crabs for legal size and return spawning females back into the water.

Of course, we would also troll for tailor in the channel, catch whiting off the sand banks, cobblers in the shallow weed beds, and bream and mulloway off the bridge at night. Uncle Ted and Aunty Eve loved their fishing and were very patient and always encouraging. I did disappoint them dreadfully once when I had something big on my line and was slowly hauling it in. It seemed to take forever, and all eyes were on me in anticipation. There was an audible gasp from Aunty Eve as we all sighted the fish as it was within mere feet of the boat. It was the biggest flounder that I had ever seen, but I lost my composure and tried to get it on board too quickly. With a brisk flick of the tail, the flounder threw the hook and disappeared back into the water. It was too much for Aunty Eve, she was so disappointed. I got a lecture on how I should have brought it to the side of the boat gently, and that she could have helped with one of the crab scoop nets to recover the fish. She wouldn't let it go and I felt bad for days. Somehow, I had let the whole side down. She may have been disappointed for me, but I suspect gastronomically she knew what we all had missed out on and she was disappointed for herself. It was a big driver in my life to not let anyone down like that again.

****

When not on any of the big holidays, our family and the Martins would troll for chopper tailor at Peppermint Grove on the Swan River. Nev was the best at catching cobblers. I never liked them because of the poisonous spike on their heads. Nev would catch them with a gidgee, a spear with three sharpened and barbed pieces of heavy gauge steel strapped to the end of a broom handle. After dark, we used to put a Tilley lamp over the bow of the boat and smash garfish. The garfish would be attracted to the light. Most floated quietly on the surface of the water, but some were jumping out of the water trying to escape predators. Sometimes we would get lucky and they would jump into the boat. We would take it in turns to stand up on the bow of the boat while someone else would be quietly rowing. It was great sport apart from the reward of eating the fish later.

Here's a funny thing, although Dad made the boat, the unofficial skipper of the boat was Uncle Ted. His contribution to the boat was to supply the outboard motor. He didn't go overboard on that contribution. He supplied a British Anzani 1.5 horsepower, hardly the most powerful outfit out there. He was a big man, ten years older than Milton, very commander like, and definite in his ideas, never backward in expressing them. He knew how to change out propellers with their split pins, and how to change oily spark plugs better than Milton, so I guess it was just a natural outcome. But I do admire the magnanimity of my father in accepting the subordinate role. Mind you he would have been so grateful for the support of Ted and Eve in managing my Mum's mood swings. Without any proof, I suspect he may also have had a bit of a flame for Aunty Eve.

If the fish weren't biting, we'd always go prawning on one of the sandy stretches of the Swan River instead. Ted and Milton would know the best places, and they would drag a prawn net parallel to the shore and then turn to shore and empty the sock of its contents. Hazel, Eve, and us kids would help sort the prawns from the sea weed and then catch and throw the prawns into big pots. Back in those days you were allowed to have a little fire on the beach, so we had many feasts on the Swan River. Our life back then revolved around the water.

12

GIVE ME THAT OLD TIME RELIGION

Mum was determined to develop my hair in the image of my father. He had wavy hair that he simply brushed straight back. It looked terrific on him, but his wave was more like a close-knit crinkle that lay flat and followed the contour of his scalp. I just didn't have the right amount of keratin and my hair stuck up like I had stuck my finger in a toaster. On the upside, I looked taller, but it gave me an image of being frightened. It was another good issue over which to have a fight with Robbie.

'Mum, why can't I have a crew cut like Graeme?' I asked. Graeme had one of those GI flat tops that looked real cool.

'I can't have you going around looking so common,' she responded.

'Why do I have to go to Sunday school? Robbie and Graeme don't have to go.'

'They are just going to miss out on the best friend in this world that you could possibly have.'

'Who is that?'

'Well, Jesus of course, you silly duffer. You're never going to know him if you don't go to Sunday school.'

I would have Sunday morning walks to the fledgling Floreat Park Methodist Church along the same road, 'The Boulevarde,' as I did to school. I never told Mum but I didn't mind because it took me past Daisy's house and she used to go as well. I never quite understood why it was so important for me because Dad, Mum, and Brian never went to church. Mum was Methodist, but for her, religion was a private affair and it was also part of her non-engagement with the community that she didn't go to the church. Dad was a nominal

Anglican and I was told that there was no Anglican church nearby. I swallowed the line. Part of the parental approach was to leak half-truths to children.

Some of the stories they told you in Sunday school were better than the ones you heard in regular school. You got to know them all because you would hear them over, and over, and over again. Things were rough back in biblical times. There were floods, fire, burning bushes with animals stuck in them, famine, plague, and disease but God was on top of it all, so you knew that everything would be alright in the end. Some of them were unbelievable. There was Noah's Ark, David and Goliath, Jonah getting swallowed by a whale. Abraham loved God so much that he was going to burn his son Isaac as an offering to God. There was also the story of Daniel in the Lion's Den, Samson and Delilah, and of course Adam and Eve. Moses floating down the Nile on a reed raft and being discovered by the Pharaoh's daughter was one of my favourites. And also when Moses grew up and parted the Red Sea so that the Israelites could escape the Egyptians.

I knew girls could be dangerous because of my experiences with Daisy, and this was all but confirmed at Sunday school. Definitely don't let them cut your hair and watch out if they hand you an apple.

The other thing I liked about Sunday school was the strident hymn music. The hymns were all sung so heartily, everything was so definite, no room for questions or confusion. Firm chords separated by running notes with simple harmonies triumphantly overcoming adversity and admonishing sin. Hymns like 'Onward Christian Soldiers', 'Soldiers of Christ, Arise', 'Am I Soldier of the Cross', 'Stand Up, Stand Up for Jesus', and 'The Strife is Over, the Battle Done' appealed to my angry, pugilistic nature. There was a war on against sin and I was prepared to take up arms. I believed most things had to be settled with a fight.

Mum had knitted me a jumper that had a coat of arms-like lion on the front. The lion was standing on his hind legs with front legs and claws extended, ready to take on anything. Born a Leo, I thought I was Richard the Lionheart off to the crusades. War, pirate, and western movies were a part of my educational intake as well.

Brian was all kitted out in a cadet army uniform and very proud of it as well. No wonder we were such a militant society.

There were other hymns about love and the love of Jesus like 'All Things Bright and Beautiful,' 'Jesus Loves Me, the Bible Tells Me So!' and 'What A Friend We Have in Jesus.' These hymns made you feel good in a different, soft way much like holding hands with Daisy.

The only time I can remember Mum and Dad coming to church was when I was presented with my own special bible. It had a navy-blue cover and was awfully thick. The words were very small, set on thin rice paper. What was most memorable was the beautiful smell that exuded when you opened it, like perfume or burning incense. No other books smelled quite like Bibles, which is all part of the mystery and the religious experience I guess. And to think Graeme and Robbie were missing out on all this. Mum and Dad beamed because I was now on the road to redemption.

13

THE DANGER OF THREE SEATER LOUNGES

Hazel had come from a large family, the Powers. She had five sisters and one brother. Pa Power was Perth's leading butcher, and the success was no accident. He selected the location of the shop for maximum trade after observing the flow of people streaming to and from the railway station to various parts of the city. Pa Power was a rags-to-riches story of great proportions. Brought up in Kalgoorlie he became the head of the family when his father left to make his fortune in South Africa and as the eldest he took on the responsibility of providing for them. There was no time to complete his schooling. He started selling lemonade down in the mines and in the brothels in his early teens. He was both street and savvy smart, he knew business and he knew how to make money.

When it came to his turn to be a parent, he tried to give his children a leg up in life, so Mum therefore had a privileged upbringing. She was brought up in a large house in Mt. Lawley complete with a tennis court. She was the third eldest child and Eve, to whom she was the closest with, was just one year older than her. Each of the girls received a good fine arts education learning the piano and how to paint. I have inherited some of Mum's wonderful paintings but am so saddened when I look at them now that I realise she just abandoned the skill at eighteen and never painted again because of her long going battle with mental illness. Aunt Eve, on the other hand, resumed her painting once her children had grown up and produced some great work and held exhibitions in Perth.

I never met Ma Power as she passed away when Mum was only fourteen years old. In the final year of Ma Power's life, Mum was told by Pa that she had to finish school in order to stay home and help her mother with all the domestic chores and assist with her convalescence. This was tough on her. She had a great mind, but she was being denied the opportunity to expand it due to family circumstances. She never spoke about these days to me, but I know she was forever bitter about her lost opportunity of having a full education.

She also gained work experience while young, counting money and providing change. She would sit up in a small caged room above the big butcher shop floor where the team of butchers were serving the public. The customers would pay for the meat and if change was required, which was normally the case, the butcher would put the money and the docket in a metal canister and by pulling a cord, the canister would fly along a wire up to where Mum sat in the treasury cage. She would remove the money and docket, do the arithmetic and mark the little sum on the docket, place it back in the canister with the correct change, ring a bell, and pull her own cord to send the canister flying back to the butchers. There were several of these trapezes connecting the shop floor to the treasury nest, and it was a mesmerizing sight to see the activity of flying canisters on a busy day. It was like being in an aviary.

Pa Power remarried and I knew his new wife as Aunty Betty. The stepmother was not well received by the five sisters, which was a sad thing given Pa Power's generosity. As a result, I did not see very much of them. He was a gregarious, happy, openhearted man. My fondest memory is having been dropped off at his apartment during a time of one of Mum's breakdowns. This was unusual because I would normally go to Ma and Pa Harrison. He was a short, dapper man often dressed in hat, waist-coat, and a fob watch on a chain with an umbrella. I needed bucking-up, so he took me for a walk. He took my hand and broke out into song;

'You and me, can we be partners
You and me, can we be friends.'

We skipped along and sang nonstop in the rain, walking around and around the block. By the time we made it back to his apartment I had forgotten all about the unreal, dreadful row that Mum and

Dad had, and the insanity that I had observed. For me at that time, he was the greatest guy on Earth.

The Powers were a diverse group of people rather than one big happy family but they did know how to party. In contrast, the Harrison family was much less outspoken and volatile as Dad only had one sister, Joy. We were all gathered at Aunt Dianne's, Mum's younger sister, Mt. Lawley house for my cousin Susan's confirmation and first communion party. The wider Power family comprised fourteen adults and eighteen children. Sadly, Pa Power and Aunty Betty were not present. Most of the children were banished to the backyard and the adults mixed inside. Our only entry to the adult world was through performances at the big parties. By performance I mean the parties became a sort of family Eisteddfod. All the children would be lined up to perform a song, dance, or play a piece on the piano.

Susan's party was going on like all other parties, that was until Uncle Alan had pulled one of his moments. The party started in the early afternoon after the full Church of England service. It was a quiet tentative start because so many of the group were forced to face their inner demons, quite unsettling for many, none more so than Uncle Alan. He preferred to not think about religion at all and to just have a good time. He especially liked being the big kid that played pranks with the children. While the adults were inside partying and singing around the piano, Alan was with the children playing hide and seek, organising egg and spoon races, and all sorts of other things. The trouble was that this was all interspersed with frequent glasses of beer. Initially his pranks with the children were quite mild, just the eccentric tripping up of some of the children in the egg and spoon races to even out results and prizes so that every child could enjoy success.

It was now about 5 PM and Uncle Alan had long since overcome the discomfort of all that religious "mumbo-jumbo." He had a large group of us gathered around a table showing us card tricks. He had our full attention.

'Who would like to earn sixpence?' he asked.

'Yes, yes!' we all responded.

'Well,' he said, 'this is what you have to do. See this full glass of water. Anyone who can put the sixpence on their forehead, hold it there for a moment, and then tilt their head forward so that it can fall in the glass gets to keep it.' Alan called the oldest child forward. 'Come over here Doug and show them how it is done.' It was not an easy thing to do even for an aware adult, let alone a child, since the top of the glass was quite small. After many attempts and some help by Uncle Alan, Doug walked off really pleased with himself and a sixpence.

'Who's next?' asked Alan.

'Me, me, me!' we all chorused, pumping our hands in the air and pushing forward.

'Dennis, come here lad. You can be next,' he said. I started trying to get the sixpence in the glass. On about the sixth attempt, Alan could see that I was tiring from the game so while I had the sixpence balancing on my forehead and eyes skyward he stretched the elastic on my shorts and poured the cold glass of water down my shorts. I was in shock. I thought I had wet myself and broke down crying. I called out at the top of my voice, 'Mum, Mum, Uncle Alan wet me pants.'

Aunty Glenda, Uncle Alan's wife, rushed outside and rose to her full height, assisted with high stiletto heels, and gave Alan a right old dressing down. 'Get a hold of yourself Alan. Just go inside will you and keep away from the children.'

A disgraced and forlorn Uncle Alan walked into the lounge room. Not all were involved in the music around the piano. Some of the more serious folk were engaged in conversation, amongst which were Uncle Ted and a friend of the family. These two had been rivals since childhood with totally different political views, and they didn't hold anything back or step down in a debate. The only seat Alan could see was on the three-seater lounge between Ted and the friend, so he sat down between them. As I was inside by now, receiving a new pair of pants from my cousin's supply, I saw the whole event evolve before me.

'Hey lads, how do you think Subiaco will go against Claremont next weekend?' Uncle Alan asked, trying to get into the conversation.

'Probably win,' Ted said before immediately continuing to talk across him. 'Trouble with you Socialists, you want to be looked after from cradle to grave.'

'What do you think?' Alan asked to Ted's friend.

'What, what?'

'Do you think Subiaco will win?'

'Oh yeah, of course. Now listen Ted, you Tories believe in this phantom trickle-down theory, let the economy rip and bugger the consequences on the environment.'

'Oh fine, and you have your hand out for the next government benefit. Where's your pride man?' Ted asked.

'I've paid taxes all my life. It's my turn to get something back. I deserve that.'

'Listen mate... ever thought you've only contributed enough tax to just fix up that small bit of bitumen outside your small house in Everton Park once in your lifetime. Not to mention the freeloading you're doing on the national health system.'

The two were talking over Uncle Alan, ignoring him. Alan thought, *I'll show these buggers,* so he would deliberately lean forward and back in a coordinated manner when they would do so to engage eye contact with each other. The result was that the three of them looked like Jews praying at the Wailing Wall.

'You see what that mining company is doing off the shore of Cape Leeuwin; they are going to destroy those precious fishing grounds you know.'

'Yeah, that mining company will make profits, employ people, and pay taxes that will help pay for your free national health. Bloody shame isn't it?' Uncle Ted responded, his eyes bloodshot.

Uncle Alan finally just snapped and stood up quickly, spilling a whole bowl of peanuts onto the floor while saying, 'You two can get lost, I can't handle any more of this shit.' He walked off.

Uncle Alan's oldest son, now in his twenties, came to save his father.

'Listen Dad, behave yourself will you. You're in real big trouble with Mum. Go over there and don't upset anyone else.'

Over there was another one of Aunt Dianne's three-seater lounges with Aunt Olive up one end and Mum down the other. There were no other spare seats so Uncle Alan had to sit in between the girls.

'Hi girls, party going well?' Alan asked.

'Yes, Alan. Listen Olive, you just don't get it. It's respect, that's what it is. Respect for God and respect for each other.'

'Oh, it's okay for you Hazel. You hide behind all that belief of yours. Live in a fantasy world you do, just dreaming.'

'Olive, you've only ever believed in the holy dollar. You should try believing in the one true holy God instead. You wouldn't have all those problems of yours if you did,' Mum replied.

At this point, Aunt Olive slapped down a large bowl of cherries on Uncle Alan's lap. It connected with a softer, more sensitive part of his anatomy. Alan bounced to his feet and yelped, 'You bloody sisters! You've always been the same.' The cherries spilled onto the carpet and Alan doubled over in pain. Stiletto-heeled Aunt Glenda rushed to the scene. 'Alan, Alan,' she said, her voice rising in pitch. 'We are going home now, give me the keys. I just can't take you anywhere.'

The party broke up quickly after the exit of Aunt Glenda, Uncle Alan, and family.

Dad could see lessons in everything for us boys, so as we drove off Dad asked us, 'Now boys, let this be a lesson to you in life. If you want to get along with people, never discuss religion and politics. What did you learn Dennis?'

'Never to trust Uncle Alan, Dad.'

'What about you, Brian?'

Brian, ever the quiet one in the family replied, 'Never sit down on a three-seater lounge between two people, Dad.'

14

LIFE AFTER DEATH

We had a big backyard with ducks, not chooks, up on the back fence. The ducks had reduced their yard to a mud bath which had a nauseating stench. The backyards back then were so large that you could get away with it but Milton never got away with it with Hazel.

'Why couldn't you have chooks like everyone else?' Mum asked.

'I wanted to try something different, Haze.'

'You're a damned fool. The ducks smell and bring in flies.'

'But Haze, don't you know that's why you win the best sponge award at the Power parties. The duck eggs are so rich.'

Dad normally had a great crop of vegetables if the ducks didn't escape their yard to destroy them. He had grape vines growing along a fence line as well as apricot, plum, almond, and mulberry trees with a cape gooseberry vine around the water tank. The mulberry tree was terrific to climb on, but when the fruit was ripe you could get your clothes in an awful mess. It meant, however, that Brian and I could keep silk worms and feed them the leaves.

We had a very busy gander and it was hard to keep the duck population under control. There came a point in time where Mum and Dad put a concerted effort towards thinning them out, and we were having roast duck every Sunday for weeks on end. The routine was to kill the duck on the Saturday and take it to the boiler in the laundry. The duck would sit in the boiling water and, with gloves on our hands, Mum and I would pluck all the feathers off. The duck would then be transferred to the refrigerator prior to cooking it up for the Sunday roast. Dad's job was to kill the duck.

Every Saturday I would keep a close eye on Dad as to the likely timing of his beheading of the duck. He had a routine that he had established so that it would give me time to go and fetch as many of my playmates around the suburb to come and witness the killing of the duck because it was quite an event. I would always go and get Robbie first and then Keith around the corner. Once I even managed to get Daisy to come and watch. That was a grand day.

Mum had an old-fashioned clothes line consisting of three separate strands of wire connected to timber T-piece posts on either side of the yard. But here's the thing: the yard had a small slope on it from right to left. Dad would chop the head off the duck just out of sight of us kids, and then tie it up by the legs on one of the wires on the high side post of the clothes line. Because of my efforts he had a grand audience. Well, the duck would flick and squirm for about thirty seconds after death due to muscle memory which would cause it to migrate down the line towards the low side post. It was certainly a macabre sight for a child.

I leaned over to Daisy and whispered in her ear, 'I think this is what Miss Harvey means about life after death.'

She looked at me all pale and sweaty and said, 'Thanks for having me over. I think I'll go home now if you don't mind.'

I replied, 'I'll walk you home.'

'Thanks.'

'We'll be able to tell Miss Harvey tomorrow that we know all about life after death. We've witnessed it. She'll be real pleased.'

15

CRICKET LESSONS

Uncle Ted taught me all I needed to know about cricket. He would spend hours with Graeme and I and show us wonderful stuff all wrapped up with lots of philosophy. It all made sense to me, so I never questioned the truth of what he was teaching.

By the time he was teaching us he wasn't a young man, so after every few balls he would take a break and give us his gems of wisdom.

'The game's played out in the centre lads. Stories are told on the sidelines. It's up to you to decide what game you want to play. And it all starts from building a strong defence,' he'd tell us.

Uncle Ted had his moment in the sun as a first-class cricketer in the Western Australian 'A' grade competition. He never bragged about it, but I just knew he had earned the right to teach us. He had been a left-hand opening batsman and a right-hand leg break or wrist spinner. I moulded myself on his teachings and became an opening batsman that could bowl 'leggies.' The only thing different was that I batted right-handed and, oh yes, I never played with Bradman in an Australian eleven against the Poms. I did, however, have some success at lower levels and shared his passion for the game.

'It's all in the footwork lads. Judge the length quickly and make your decision to either play forward or back. Once you are committed, that's it. Either watch the ball onto the bat or let it go.'

He would demonstrate how little of the stumps are visible around the bat when it is held in front of them. When you look at it like that, you realise how hard it is for the bowler. You can let a lot of balls pass through to the wicketkeeper.

'You are the opening batsman. You are there to see the new ball fast bowlers off, tire them out, make them despondent, and protect the rest of the side from the best bowlers. They really get pissed off when they run flat out towards you and let the ball fly while you just protect your stumps and let the ball go. They hate it and it's your job to break their spirit. Once you've done that, you can make runs and so can the rest of the team.'

'Good footwork allows you to alter the length of the ball that is bowled. You can use your whole crease.' And he would demonstrate how far forward you could come with the forward defensive stroke and how far back you could go with the backward defensive stroke.

'Get in behind the ball. It is easier to avoid being hit by doing that, and you have a second line of defence, your pads.'

I soon realised the wisdom of that lesson while playing with Robbie. You can pick the unskilled batsman; they back off to square leg against fast bowlers to avoid being hit. Their fear is there for all to see and the bowler can then intimidate them. Often, they will be hit as they step into trouble. A hard ball coming at you at 100 kph can be intimidating. Uncle Ted and I played our cricket at a time when there was minimal protective gear and definitely no helmets. It demanded that you learn correct technique.

'Scoring runs is secondary; it's all about survival. Your wicket is sacrosanct. You cannot influence the game when you are out watching from the sidelines.'

I had heard that one so many times before.

'Play with a straight bat. To get the correct line, you point the elbow of your leading, upper arm on the bat at the ball.'

'Never hit the ball in the air, it's just another way to get out.'

To learn that lesson, he would have us bat one-handed. The controlling hand is the upper hand on the bat, the power hand is the lower hand.

'Observe the control you have,' he would say. 'The left hand and elbow can direct the vertical blade in any direction and allow the pushing of a single into the gaps in the field. The blade on impact is facing down towards the ground and the ball is therefore hit down, not up. It's a great way to survive as an opening batsman if you are down the other end, so pushing these little singles is essential as the two of you rotate the strike. The bowler has to think of a different strategy and cannot intimidate you.'

There was so much to take in when you were with him. I absorbed all his training, and one Christmas I received the Ken Meuleman cricket book. The book contained several photos displaying all the cricket shots and how to hold the ball for different bowling styles. In a full-length mirror I would try and replicate the correct position to play the shots.

16

THE ART OF CRICKET
BY EDMUND MARTIN

It was a hot Sunday and the Martins had come over from their North Perth home to have dinner with us; roast duck, of course. They had come early for a mid-afternoon swim at nearby City Beach to cool off. The waves were rolling into the shore in sets, separated by large three- metre high waves. To Graeme and me, these were both great challenges and frightening. None of us had surfboards but we could all body surf. The skill was to select the right wave and catch it at just the right time so that you didn't get dumped. When a large wave came in between the regularly spaced sets, the idea was to swim towards it before it broke and dive under and through the wave. The trouble was you wouldn't always get it right and mistakes tended to hurt. You could get caught up, unceremoniously dumped in a whirlpool of sand and sudsy water, then bounced along the bottom. You had to have a good lung full of air and last the distance until the wave dissipated on the shoreline.

I had just experienced a bad dump and churn, so I made my way back to shore. Uncle Ted was already there, sitting under an umbrella sucking on an orange.

'How's your cricket going?' he asked.

'I am Captain of the Floreat Park Primary School eleven, Unc,' I told him as I stuck my chest out like I was some sort of hero. 'I was last man out in the last match and I took three for fifteen bowling fast.'

'That's great, Dennis. I think you're ready for the spin bowling lesson now.'

'The spin bowling lesson?' I repeated.

'Yes. You want to forget that fast bowling nonsense. Waste of time, waste of space. The real art is in the spin bowling and playing against it. It's the ultimate game of cut and thrust like playing chess or fencing.'

Arriving back home, Graeme and I hustled Uncle Ted to come play cricket out in the backyard. Brian and Nev went away and did their own thing. They were into dinky toy model cars. I could never accumulate them. Whenever I received a good one as a present, Brian would do some outlandish trade of goods and I seemed to end up with next to nothing and he walked away with my best cars. Seven years is a big gap in understanding the art of negotiation. Dad stayed inside helping Mum and Aunty Eve with dinner preparations. Unc didn't have to be asked twice.

'So boys, let's assume you've seen the fast bowlers off. Now you have to face the spin bowlers. Right, you first Dennis. I'll bowl a few down and see what you make of them,' Uncle Ted said.

Well, I couldn't hit any of his balls. They would break off in different directions, they would swing in the air in the opposite direction to the way they would break, and just when you thought you were at the ball, the ball would drop on you and not be where it was supposed to. I had never seen anything like it in my life.

'Your turn Graeme.'

And the same thing happened to Graeme. This was a complete revelation, a new art to us both.

'Okay boys, now my turn. Bowl a few balls down to me Dennis.'

Since my latest figures were three for fifteen bowling fast for Floreat Park Primary School, I gave Uncle Ted the best I had. He batted them away with disdain, some of them one handed, and he even batted one handed with his non-dominant right hand. I was soon exhausted trying to bowl fast, so I threw the ball to Graeme to see if he could do any better. Uncle Ted then demonstrated how to use your feet to dance down the wicket.

'See boys? You see the technique. You can skip down the wicket by taking two paces quickly and smother the spin of the ball. That's the way to play a spin bowler because you cannot always determine which way it will break out of the hand. You can get down the wicket at least six feet this way. If the spin bowler bowls any shorter than that, you can safely play back, and you have plenty of time to play the ball off the wicket.'

He then showed us the different ways you could grip the ball to bowl both wrist and finger spinners. He was a master wrist spinner.

'The key is to have flexible, oily wrists,' he explained.

We both sat on the grass before him, mesmerised.

'You see, the leg break comes out of the front of the hand, the googly or wrong-un comes out of the back of the hand with the same action but instead of rotating clockwise it's now rotating anti-clockwise. The googly will therefore swing in the air towards the off and then break towards the leg side, like a regular off break bowler. The standard leg spin ball will swing in the air towards the leg and break towards the off side. That should be your stock ball. Then, with the same action, you can bowl a top spinner by changing your wrist to be between the two extremes of leg spin and googly. The ball spins vertically on its axis and sucks down quickly, and it will fall short of where the batsman expects it and he, if he's not careful, will be suckered into hitting the ball in the air. Right-oh, have a go yourselves.'

I stepped up to the plate. First efforts at spin bowling can be atrocious.

'Let's just bowl off a half-length pitch for a start, boys. Dennis, what's this skip before your delivery stride? You don't need that. You don't need a long run up and you don't need that skip,' Uncle Ted said.

I never bowled fast from that day forth. I attempted to become a spin bowler just like Uncle Ted. I have had a lifetime to reflect that the skip just before the delivery stride, that I had naturally developed and discovered as a youngster, was just like the one used by Dennis Lillee many years later. Some nights I toss and turn and dream of what may have been.

Hot and sticky, we three then joined everyone else for roast duck and my favourite dessert, bread and butter pudding. Graeme and I retreated to bed to make up some stories, and the adults played bridge well into the wee hours of the morning.

****

Not many weekends would pass before we would be over at the Martins for dinner. It would be their turn to reciprocate, and the cricket lessons would continue in Uncle Ted's backyard. Later in the night, Uncle Ted and Aunty Eve, if requested, would put on a concert. Uncle Ted was a fine violinist and Aunt Eve would accompany him on the piano. Oh, it was grand to see him tuck the violin into his chin and dramatically strike the first note of Mozart's Adagio in E Major. Playing the violin is drama and theatre. It cannot be simply played, it is a performance. His bow would fly back and forth; the odd note dramatically struck would dislodge a strand of his thinning hair which he would attempt to restore to its rightful place with a re-tuck of the instrument into his neck and a flick of his head. There were times when he would pluck the strings with his fingers and other times when he would strike the strings such that the bow would quickly bounce up and down whilst holding the same chord. What a sound that would produce. I believe that nothing can quite match solo violin music. There is a performance grandeur provided by the theatre and a physicality to bow strike, bow angle, and delicate finger work that no other instrument can provide. Alas, my musicality went in a different direction into the brass world. Lord, when I return, could I have a go at the violin?

That night at the performance, although so young, I made the connection of playing the violin with cricket. Uncle Ted batted as a violinist, intelligently, with finesse, subtlety, and mastery. The way he batted was no less art than playing the violin.

When reaching the age of one hundred in September 2002, 'The West Australian' newspaper took him down to the WACA ground and took a photo of him in front of the score board with one hundred not out against his name. To take the photo, they had him standing on a wooden box. His son, Nev, himself in his seventies, told me, 'It was blowing a gale and I was holding his legs out of sight of the camera so that the old fella wouldn't fall off the box.' The photo showed Uncle Ted whimsically smiling through his poorly shaved whiskers with a cricket ball held aloft, showing off his leg spinner grip. Aside from his six seasons in A-grade pennant cricket for Subiaco and Mt Lawley he only had two first class appearances, one for Western Australia and one in an Australian eleven, both against England in 1932/33. Back in those days, the English touring side would land in Freemantle and play a WA representative side. Due to its isolation from the eastern states WA was not then a part of the Sheffield Shield interstate competition.

1932/33 was the year of the Bodyline series, led by Jardine along with the terror fast bowler Larwood. This tour by England was to become the most controversial tour series in Test history. Bodyline was a strategy of bowling short of a length to a packed leg side field, and it was concocted by the Poms to counter the brilliance of Don Bradman. Larwood played in the first game against WA, but this was kept under wraps in the Combined Australian eleven game as the English didn't want Bradman to see Larwood until the test matches began. Uncle Ted, however, reported that he was roughed up with leg side bowling and fielders by the fast bowler Brian Bowes. 'It was a disease. They gave me a bit of it. I received a couple of whacks. You only wore pads, gloves, and a box in those days, and the box wasn't much good. I got hit and had a bruise an inch and a half long,' he told 'The West Australian' reporter John Townsend.

Uncle Ted was a mature club bowler when he was picked to play against the touring England team. They couldn't overlook him as he had topped the A grade pennant bowling averages in the two previous seasons. At that stage, he had not developed his batting as well as his bowling. In the first game, playing for WA, he took six wickets for one hundred and sixty- eight runs over the two innings, three for one hundred and eighteen in the first, and three for fifty in the second. He claimed the wickets of Sutcliffe, the Nawab of Paturdi and Wyatt, a distinguished group of players. In the second match, the representative Australian eleven included Don Bradman and Vic Richardson. Unfortunately, Ted took no wickets in that match and was plastered all over the ground with the abysmal figures of none for one hundred and twenty-six. This would have broken a weaker man.

Years later I asked him, 'Tell me about the ball that got Sutcliffe, Unc.'

He responded, 'I finally got one on a length. Now that's the truth. Some prick journo wrote up my performance after the second match as Martin showed a lot of variety. He interspersed full tosses with long hops. Maybe Sutcliffe just got tired.'

'Don't sell yourself short, Unc. The records show you beat him with a well flighted googly. In my eyes, you were the precursor of Shane Warne. What happened to your bowling after 1933?' I asked. 'You seemed to lose the magic.'

'Look, there was a symbiotic relationship with my violin playing and spin bowling. Playing the violin gave me very flexible wrists. I sprained my wrist replacing that rotten fence down the back of our North Perth house. I was never the same after that, so I concentrated on my batting. Eventually, I became a grafting opening batsman that could handle difficult conditions, and there were plenty of bad wickets back then. My technique allowed me to survive when others were failing.'

Uncle Ted taught me cricketing technique, sure, but he also taught me so much more. He gave me courage. It takes enormous courage to face up to the fastest bowling that a side can throw at you when they are at their freshest and most optimistic; before they are broken. You can receive some nasty blows when you get your timing wrong. All of that is one thing, but it dwarfs in comparison to the courage required to be a wrist spinner. It is the most difficult of arts to master. Like a beautiful woman or a strip tease artist that promises so much, there can be dramatic disappointment. Like a bipolar sufferer, the exponent can ride huge highs and massive lows. It's a high roller risky game and you are a tease to the captain. He knows that if you get it right you can win a game, get it wrong though and you may well have cost him the game. The exponent has to believe in themselves because the margin between being absolutely brilliant and bowling unplayable balls, to the worst and most expensive rubbish balls that are punished all over the park, is so small.

Uncle Ted was a wrist spinner, WA's best for two seasons. He lived on the edge with enormous courage and gave it his all. What else can anyone ask for?

I added Uncle Ted to the list of people I could not let down when I stepped onto the cricket field and the field of life.

17
MENTAL ILLNESS

One day out of the blue Daisy asked me, 'So what does your Dad do?

'He's a public servant. Why do you want to know?'

'My Mum said it would be good to know.'

'Did she really?'

'Yep. She said I can't play with just anyone. So, what's he do?'

'He works at the Attorney General's Department.'

'What's that?'

'Well they've got generals, so it must be a special part of the army I suppose.'

'Really? But I haven't seen him in a uniform.'

'Well no. He's too important to wear a uniform.'

'How about a game of hopscotch?'

'Sounds good to me.'

If anyone asked about his job, Dad had given me my running instructions. And I had replied to the letter apart from the army embellishment; that was all my own creativity. It would be many years later when I would discover that he worked for ASIO, the Australian Security Intelligence Organisation, as an intelligence officer. He had worked in intelligence in the army during the war and, like so many of his fellow officers, was recruited for ASIO because of his wartime experience. It had been impressed upon me not to talk about any of this secret stuff.

Dad would take trips over to Melbourne, Canberra, and Sydney. It was a big deal back then. A part of his job was to go to cocktail parties, entertain, and develop contacts. He was a party animal and liked that role but given Mum's instability, it wasn't easy. She was like an eccentric artist that could say or do something outlandish on a whim. But it was worse than that because there were moments of insanity. We could all see it coming. Emotional pressure would build and build until the cooker could take no more of it. The lid would fly off and the clean up afterwards was always messy.

From my perspective, Dad's life looked like a series of apologies followed by ceaseless recoveries. The white lies would just flow without any effort from his lips, but his heart was torn asunder after each stormy episode, after each disappointment and embarrassment. The drama was so intense that I would question how he could possibly go on. Why doesn't he run away, leave her? She was holding his career back. He rejected promotions and new postings, some of which could have taken the family overseas. Brian and I observed the pattern. Mum would return to a semblance of good health and Dad would start negotiations. He would talk her to a point of accepting a new life and a possible move, but she couldn't hold to a decision. She would second guess, get nervous, and change her mind. They should have called the big dipper at Luna Park "The Hazel Ride."

Towards each emotional crisis Mum would retreat further into her shell and start reading the Bible more frequently. She obviously thought the answers were to be found within, if only you could work them out. It was so cryptic. Then she would consult all the wrong people. She would run to Aunt Lucy, one of her younger sisters. Aunt Lucy had been let down early on in her life when her husband left her along with two young children so that he could become a movie star in Hollywood. I, along with my seventeen cousins, was taken to the movies to see him in the movie Long John Silver. He didn't have any lines and you had to look closely in order to see him in one of the scenes. His name did come up in the credits at the end of the movie. It was the highlight of Aunt Lucy's life, and she lived in the hope of his return. We suspect it was the peak of his career as well. We never saw him again. After that disappointment, Aunt Lucy took her solace in the Bible. So naturally she felt she could help Mum when emotional turmoil beset her. The pairing never helped a family resolution, but the two of them did feel closer to God.

Not letting yourself and others down in life came through in my upbringing driven by my silent observations rather than any verbal instruction. The reality is that nobody lives up to the image they have of themselves, and nobody is as good or as bad as you imagine. My father was my protector, not my mother. He shielded me from the worst of my mother's excesses and encouraged me to excel. There was stability there for a start, a constancy of representation and performance. I knew what to expect from him. With Mum, there were just too many surprises. Men sort of remain the one person, don't they? For a start, they don't wear makeup. But women present so many different images to the world. There is the made-up image full of lipstick, mascara, and powder but when that's all gone, and you see them daily without the external pretence, there is someone else. There is a dichotomy, a lack of consistency in that. A developing child must learn to process that. Have psychologists examined this aspect of our social development? Perhaps it would prove to be a worthy field of research.

18

THWARTED MUSICAL AMBITIONS

When I was only about six years old, Robbie's latest dare was billycart racing. Everything fun seemed to involve some form of danger. The best billycart run was down Orrel Avenue. The downhill Orrel Avenue run hit the Birkdale cross street, and at the other side of the T-intersection was the kindergarten playground where I started my fighting a few years earlier. We would take it in turns to race down the footpath across Birkdale Street, and the run would be broken by the grass at the Kindergarten.

We would take turns as spotter for the cars coming along Birkdale Street. If a car was coming it was the responsibility of the spotter to raise a red flag, and if the run had already started it had to be aborted. The brakes on these billycarts were next to useless; pull a wooden leaver that would apply a stick with a bit of leather strapped to it at the rear ball bearing wheels. It was safer to swerve violently right into Mrs Macintosh's hedge as opposed to using that brake. If you missed her hedge you hit the rose bushes and that could be painful. Not only that, it could mean the end of billycarting for the day because Mrs MacIntosh would come out and tell us to clear off.

Robbie seemed to have a different concept of the proximity of a car approaching than I did. It took me awhile to realise that he was playing with my life. I knew his dad could fix things but bloody Flood Plumbing wasn't going to put me together again if something went wrong. My ultimate excuse was that Dad hasn't fixed the cart yet.

Quick as a flash Robbie would say, 'You can use mine.'

'Nope. I can't handle yours. The steering's wonky.'

'You're a pussy.'

'No, I'm not. Tell you what, you can try and knock my head off bowling fast if you like.'

It was shortly after one of the rose bush-aborted downhill runs that, as I was leaving from my piano lesson with Mrs. Schmidt, I thought of a plan of walking a few extra blocks before catching the bus. With the money I would save, I could buy some chips off Mr Phillips. My walk took me past the front door of the Wembley Salvation Army hall. I must have been a right sight all scabby-kneed and scabby-elbowed, but I decided to knock on the door anyway. The door opened and channelling my best Oliver Twist I asked,

'Please sir, I would like to play a musical instrument.'

'What's your name, son?'

'Dennis Harrison.'

'Well, you can call me Major Bruce, or just Major for short.'

'My father's a general, sir, with the attorney generals.'

'Is that so? Can you read music Dennis?'

'Oh yes, I play the piano real good. I learn from Mrs Schmidt up on Cambridge Street.'

The kindly man looked down on me, 'Well Dennis, I am in charge of the band and we would love to have you. Come back next Tuesday at six o'clock and we will start you on the tenor horn.'

'I like the look of the trombone, sir.'

'After a couple of years, and if you show promise, we could try you on the trombone but it is a very hard instrument for a youngster. Your arms aren't long enough yet, you wouldn't reach seventh position.'

'Oh, okay Major. The tenor horn it is then. Thank you. I'll see you next Tuesday.'

Much later of course I would understand that the tenor horn, because of its small size, is a good starter instrument for a youngster. All enthusiastic and excited I skipped home. At dinner that night I announced, 'Mum, Dad. I'm going to join the Salvation Army Band. Major Bruce can start me on the tenor horn.'

'Over my dead body you are,' my father boomed. 'No son of mine is going to join the Salvos and get all religious on me.'

I didn't understand any of the references to religion and the adopted lifestyle. I just wanted to play a musical instrument. I finished the remainder of my meal, excused myself from the table, and despondently sulked off to my bedroom.

Later, Mum came down to see me and gathered me into her bosom saying,

'You stick with your piano lessons, Dennis. You see it will all be for the best.'

I surely thought that Mum being all religious might have stuck up for me and convince Dad that it was a good opportunity for me to spread my musical wings, but I guess it wasn't meant to be. There must have been a deep underlying desire for me to play a brass instrument as I joined a brass band as a raw beginner when I was in my fifties.

This incident may have triggered my lifelong debate about the benefits or detriments of religion in life and mental health. Dad never supported, let alone accepted, Mum's need for religion. I am sure he saw it as a destructive force in her life. If a mentally unstable individual is hearing voices, it is a small step to be hearing the voice of God instructing them how to live their life. What comes first, the voice of God fleshed out in the scriptural inspiration, or the paranormal voice of the individual's mind? If Dad had allowed her greater religious freedom, been more tolerant and supportive, would she have led a happier, fulfilling life? I debate this still.

19

FIFTEEN IS A GOOD AVERAGE

One Friday night when I was in my second to last year at primary school, I remember receiving a phone call from Graeme.

'We are one short tomorrow to make up a team. Can you help us out?' Graeme asked.

'Should be able to. Where is it?'

'Wellington Square, right in the city.'

'Who's it with?'

'I've been playing in a matting competition for the North Perth Temperance League.'

'Have you?'

Neither of us spoke for a moment. This was news to me. I thought Graeme told me everything.

'Anyway, what's a Temperance League?'

'They're Presbyterians I think. They're dead against drinking alcohol.'

'You know we are Methodists, Graeme.'

'Listen, there's Methodists in the side. Besides, you know I'm nothing and I play for them. They won't even ask you.'

'Gee... I don't know.'

'If they ask you, just say you're a Presbyterian.'

'I couldn't do that. That would be lying. Dad wouldn't let me join the Salvos you know.'

'Forget the religion will you. It's only a game of cricket.'

'Okay. How do I get there?'

'Dad said to catch the number forty-five trolley bus that goes down Wellington Street. Just ask the driver to let you off at Wellington Square. Be there by nine o'clock.'

'Thanks for the invite. Looking forward to plastering some Presbyterians.'

****

This was all very new to me, coming down to this part of town by myself. Despite there being many groups of cricketers dispersed throughout the parklands, I found Graeme without too much trouble.

'I thought you weren't coming,' he said.

'The bus was a bit late,' I replied.

'We've lost the toss and East Perth is batting. I'll tell the skipper you can bowl some leggies.'

They put me at square leg. That's a position that captains love to hand out to fieldsman they know nothing about. I seemed to be one of the smallest kids on the oval. That's because I was at least two years younger than the other players. It started a trend in my junior sporting activities. In pugilistic terms, I was always fighting above my weight. Good training for life as it builds courage.

I had quite a bit of running around to do as East Perth scored one hundred and twenty-one runs. That's quite a big score for underage cricket. Then it was our turn and as I was making up the numbers and the runt of the pack I came in last when the score was nine for sixty. It was really hot. All the players and the umpires were looking forward to a quick end to the game. Graeme was still in and had already scored eighteen runs.

He came up to me as I walked clumsily to the crease with oversize pads on my legs. I had gloves on with green spiky rubber stuck to each finger. I loved the smell of the gloves.

'Give it your best shot, Dennis. Just remember all the things Dad told you. Only play the balls you have to, play with a straight bat, and keep the ball on the ground.'

I was feeling important. 'Right, no worries.'

With great theatre I boldly called out, 'Centre to centre, please Ump.'

I marked the centre point with a piece of chalk that was kept behind the stumps. The umpire had his hand held out horizontal to stop the fast bowler, who already had five wickets, from running in. I made him wait for as long as I could get away with pretending to survey where all the fieldsmen were placed, and then I took my guard. By now the fast bowler was frustrated, he ran in and gave me his fastest ball. I stepped back in my crease to protect my stumps and just let the ball fly past to the keeper. I then took a little walk to square leg while the fielding side returned the ball to the bowler. I took guard again and, repeating the move, I let the ball go through to the keeper just like Uncle Ted had told me. This was going well. The next ball was full length and on the stumps, so I played the perfect forward defensive stroke, elbow up and pointing towards the bowler, and patted it straight down the wicket.

'Over,' called the umpire.

Graeme walked down the wicket and said, 'That's the go, Dennis. Doing well. We've got to bat for an hour and fifteen minutes if we are going to save this game.'

'We can do that,' I replied.

I treated each ball as though it were a time bomb and patted it around in the Ken 'Slasher' Mackay way. I would walk down the wicket and tap the matting or remove pieces of imaginary grit from it. The longer we were out there, the easier it became. The bowling side and the umpires were becoming quite restless. These two batsmen, and this damn little kid in particular, were holding up the victory celebrations.

They never got us out and the game was drawn. I was fifteen not out and Graeme was forty-one not out. We were partners and encouraged ourselves at the end of each over. We were really chuffed and couldn't wait to get home and relate the whole story.

Graeme said to me, 'You know that walking down the wicket stuff and patting down the wicket?'

'Yeah.'

'That's what you do on turf wickets in case there is loose turf or a hole in the wicket. It doesn't mean a thing when you're playing on matting.'

'Is that right? But it uses up some time doesn't it? And it pisses off the opposition.'

He laughed, 'You're right there. I guess you're a lot smarter than I thought.'

We had done Uncle Ted proud. We had honoured all of his teachings. We didn't let him down. I played the rest of my cricketing days out in a similar manner. As an opener I would score fifteen in an hour or so, and I figured I had done my best for the side. The crowd would die of boredom and, after an hour or so of intense concentration, my brain was fried. I never won the batting averages. It's a bit hard when you average fifteen. But I never tired of breaking fast bowler's egos.

20

CHASING DAISY NIELSEN ENDS BADLY

In my last year at primary school I lost my good looks chasing Daisy Nielsen around the school yard. She pinched one of my dodgem cars as a prank.

If we weren't playing football or cricket, we boys were playing marbles or dodgem cars. I was only an average marble player but since I knew how to fight that helped whenever the inevitable dispute arose. Every boy carried their marbles around in a little homemade, cotton, string-drawn bag. Marbles are small balls of glass in a multitude of different combinations of spectacular colour and design. Some were perfectly clear while others were opaque and creamy. We gave them all sorts of different names. There were tom-bowlers, cats-eyes, agates, corkscrews, swirls, clearies, creamies, pee-wees, onion skins, and several more. They were prized possessions, and everyone had their favourites.

The wimps played friendly games where you would recover your own marbles at the end of the game, but the real game was 'keeps.' We played by drawing an approximate four-foot circle on the ground within which each player put an equal number of marbles. These marbles were at risk of being permanently lost. Each player had their taw or shooting marble and the idea was to fire it at the marbles in the ring to hit them outside the ring. If you succeeded, the taw could be recovered and the marble that had been hit outside the ring could be kept giving the player another shot. The shooting technique was to hold the marble in the crook of the index finger and with the thumb placed behind the marble to forcibly flick it forward.

The selection of your taw marble deserved great consideration. Its size and weight were important, and it was inevitably one of your favourite and most valuable marbles. Here was the rub though: if your taw marble didn't finish outside the ring on your shot, it was fair game for your opponent to fire at it and win it. You had to use a different marble then on your shot. That's why the idea was to fire your taw like a blue tongue lizard strike so, that if you didn't hit a ring marble outside the ring, at least your taw left the ring.

You can imagine how serious a game this could be. Once a real game was on there would be a large gathering of spectators surrounding the players. It was safer to be a spectator and have your bag of marbles safely tied around your belt with a hand on the bag. That way you could feel the high stakes that these brave players were up against.

Marbles was a lesson in capitalism. The real cool guys had the biggest bag of marbles and they kept winning. Once they were on top as one of the best, it was hard to be knocked off. Since they had a larger lot of marbles, those that they do put at risk would be their inferior ones put up against better quality marbles. With skill, trading smarts, and superior negotiation they would forever remain kingpins. My marble bag was only of average size. I couldn't compete with the top mobsters, so I played in the second division and chose my opponents carefully after doing the appropriate research. That way I survived. Often, I played the lower stakes dodgem cars.

Dodgem cars involved the use of modified dinky toy cars. From eight paces apart, two players would fire their dodgem cars at each other to cause them to collide. With high speed collisions the winner of the contest would be the car that remained upright. The loser would hand over the stake, normally one marble. Cars were modified by putting semi-circular roofs on them to assist in their self-righting. Modified bulldog-clips were handy for that purpose. Paperclips attached from the bottom of the car in a fan arrangement was another technique. It was good if your father was handy with a soldering iron. My Dad was, but he would often be away working so I had to fend for myself or do another bad trade with Brian to get good modifications.

It was tough on the cars and this game required a lot of running repairs. So, amongst your lunch and decaying bananas in your school bag, there had to be your marble bag and your dodgem car in its own special box. It was in the world of marbles and dodgem cars that risk, reward, enterprise, and survival lessons were taught.

****

Daisy Nielsen and her little clan of female helpers concocted this plan to steal my dodgem car. She used her best friend Janice to distract me. I thought all the girls had come to watch the contest I was having with Michael Henderson, and while he was having time out to repair his *Chevrolet* and Janice was telling me how good I was, Daisy snatched my *Ford Imperial* and ran off. I saw her do it out of the corner of my eye and by the time I rose from my cross-legged position and broke through the ring of girls, Daisy had a good fifteen metre head start. I was all up for the contest licking my lips, mouth wide open and closing fast at full speed, when suddenly Daisy came to an abrupt stop. I ploughed right ahead and implanted my front teeth in the back of her head as though biting an apple. There was blood everywhere and it wasn't Daisy's. My right front tooth was loose, and the teachers were called. I was sent home with the instructions to hold my tooth in place with my thumb and index finger.

Mum put me to bed while I continued to hold my tooth. Dad arrived home that night and after a moment of sympathy he gave me some advice. 'Dennis, girls don't always run away, sometimes they like to get caught.'

I replied, 'I'll keep that in mind, if ever there is going to be a next time.' I didn't know it then, but this was to be the most comprehensive education he was to give me about the 'birds and the bees and the cigarette trees.'

The incident didn't do much for my appearance. After a visit to the dentist, who declared that the front tooth was dead, he removed the dead nerve through a hole drilled in the back of the tooth, and I lived through my teen years with a grey front tooth. Mum was still insisting that my hair be brushed straight back, so I was an appealing sight to the opposite sex, electric hair and a grey tooth. I think I might have even frightened Robbie at that time in my life, but the sight of me was more than any girl could possibly handle. It wasn't until I was eighteen when my grey tooth was capped, and I had charge of my own hair that I thought I had a chance with girls. I was self-conscious of my appearance for all those years, not to be assisted by the onset of teenage acne, and I hid from the world by throwing myself into sport, books, and school work.

My dentist was an ex-army friend of Dads. I don't know if Dad had some special mates-rates deal with him, but he handled the drill like a carpenter doing tongue and groove joints with a router. Any sign of infection he would carve a central trough in the tooth and then trowel up the centre with amalgam. The only remnant of the tooth was at the edges. Whatever savings Dad made on dentistry, I have paid for a thousand times over throughout my life with high maintenance due to teeth breaking off and amalgam repair. Breakdowns would often occur whilst travelling. I became accustomed to the residue of amalgam and the feel of a broken tooth in my mouth. I would explore the depths of the cavity with my tongue while thinking about Dad's army dentist and Daisy, where all my troubles began.

21

PERTH MODERN SCHOOL

It was time to transition to secondary school. I was accepted into Perth Modern School in Subiaco. Perth Modern was a prestigious school that had produced many individuals who have achieved high Australian honours, including fourteen Rhodes Scholars. Some of the luminaries that had preceded me were Kim E. Beazley, Bob Hawke, H. C. 'Nugget' Coombs, and Sir Paul Hasluck. Entry until 1958 was only by scholarships that were awarded on academic achievement. After that, the school became open attendance based on regional location. I started in 1959 which is just as well since I hadn't exactly worked hard for academic achievements in primary school.

On the night before I was to start my first day at Modern, I received the best pep talk that my father had ever given me.

'Now listen up good, Dennis.' He sat down on the chair in front of me, placed his two large hands on either shoulder and looking straight into my eyes said, 'You've won the lottery, son. Over ninety percent of Perth Modern graduates go on to university. I want you to be a part of that tradition. This is your big chance in life. Grab it with both hands. You had a lot of fun at primary school, but this secondary schooling is dead serious. Make the most of it. You only get one chance. Your Mum and I didn't have such an opportunity, you know. Now I don't want to hear about any scraps or fights you are having. You respect everyone, you hear me? Work and study hard, and the world will be your oyster. Got that?'

'Yes Dad. I won't let you down.'

This was a motivational speech that I believe changed my life. In the transition to high school I had abandoned the macho bravado of a fight a day. Robbie had moved on to a technical school and then ultimately into an apprenticeship with Flood Plumbing. We now mixed in different circles and, as though somebody had flicked a switch, we adopted a more responsible persona. After Dad's speech, I was only ever in one 'physical' fight throughout my entire secondary schooling. Once you advance from 'child weighted' punches and receive the force of an adult punch and the pain incurred by both the giver and the receiver, you quickly realise that it's a mug's game. Verbal negotiation and positioning is far superior.

To get to school I had a three-mile bike ride down Salvado Road. Proficiency as a cyclist was not one of my strengths. I seemed to make a lot of bad decisions as was evident by the amount of scratches and torn clothes as a result of accidents. This disappointed Dad as he had done some competitive road cycling, so he knew how to take care of a bike. But as he was neither a good teacher nor a patient man, he hadn't handed that skill set on to me.

On weekends I played under-sixteen cricket at Floreat Park and under-sixteen football with Wembley. Again, I was one of the youngest in the sides. Gary and Robbie Flood were playing with Wembley so that was good enough for me. Under-sixteen cricket in Floreat Park was played on a turf wicket which was amazing and underlines the good development of Western Australian cricket over the years.

Out of the small primary school fish bowl and cast into the bigger competitive pool of a much larger secondary school as a new chum, my sporting prowess was yet to be discovered. I found myself batting at number eight in a school game at Perth Modern. It was also the first time I was hit in the nuts. The skipper called out to me as I was walking out to bat.

'You got a box on?'

'Nah,' I replied over my shoulder, supremely confident. 'I won't need it, they've only got the spinners on.'

'Right you are.'

Well, no sooner had I gotten out there when they brought the fast bowler back on. I got right behind the ball, just like Uncle Ted had taught me, but the bat didn't come down in time. I was caught dead centre in the crown jewels. I dropped like a sack of potatoes, the pain was excruciating. Is this how women feel in childbirth? You're about to pass out and all you hear are innocuous questions asked in great mirth, 'Are you alright mate? How are they hanging?'

'They'll eventually sort themselves out young fellow,' the teacher who was umpiring remarked. Two teammates came out onto the ground, and with my arms draped around each of their shoulders they dragged me off.

The teacher instructed them, 'Just keep him moving and walking.' I walked like one of those dolls that only have one pin in their hips and the back foot drags on the ground until it is released forward in a delayed, desultory fashion.

'Best take him home to get the Bird's Eye onto them,' said the teacher.

'The *Birds Eye*? What are you talking about?' I squeaked.

'The frozen peas. Keeps the swelling down.'

'Oh great. That will be a lovely sight for Mum,' I responded with my now high-pitched voice.

****

There were early signs of an academic future for me at Perth Modern. As I knuckled down and took an interest in school work, by the end of the first year and to everyone's amazement, the report card revealed that I was second in the class. I was strong in science, math, geography, French, and history but abysmal in technical drawing, woodwork, and metalwork. Dad responded on the report card, 'A very pleasing report. I want Dennis to do the matriculation course.' I think it was self-evident that I should do so because I wasn't going to make it in the trades with five for woodwork and four for metalwork.

Our lives were to be taken over by bigger things than mere academic results.

22

MAYBE BILLY GRAHAM CAN HELP

I knew there were big things afoot, but as the youngest I was always shielded from the worst. It was a part of the cloak of secrecy which shrouded the family. Dad had put his career on hold for a long time and had declined any promotions, desperately trying to stabilise his domestic situation. However, towards the end of 1959 Mum and Dad were in negotiations about a possible family move to Melbourne and a significant promotion for Dad. If you want a career to progress, there are only so many times you can say no. Opportunities can dry up overnight. Dad had said no many times before but must have known he was approaching his last offer. He desperately wanted to say yes.

Dad would negotiate with Mum about the move. The sands of negotiation changed all the time like peace talks in the Middle East. The trouble was that Mum could not maintain a position. Frozen with indecision like a rabbit caught in spotlights, she would vacillate with selling the family home and heading east or just staying put. Dad was driven to despair. Brian was getting married young which at least had the reward of escape from the impossible family turmoil. I received my first pair of long trousers for Brian's wedding and was taken for my first restaurant meal, Chinese. I had chicken chow mein with noodles. What else? Prior to that, any eating out was fish and chips at Freemantle or a burger with the lot at Burnie's, on the Swan River.

We were surrounded by signs of Mum's fragmentation.

'You are taking your medication, Hazel?' Dad would ask.

'Yes,' she lied.

For Mum, it was a vicious merry-go-round. Mental illness can be so debilitating and cruel. Getting the diagnosis correct is the first hurdle and the second is getting the treatment right. For Mum, they got neither right! The use of lithium for bipolar was discovered by an Australian psychiatrist, John Cade, in 1949 but it wasn't until the sixties that it became widely used. An amazing breakthrough, but one too late for Mum. She was treated with heavy mood-altering drugs that came with dire consequences. Naturally she hated these drugs. They slowed her mental faculties and made her lifeless. The Largactil kept her passive, non-violent, depressed, and non-threatening but also non-responsive and lifeless. It must have torn the heart out of her. Once she had had enough, she would fight back and stop taking the medication. Life, creativity, and fun would return for a brief window until it was replaced with mania, instability, aggression, verbal attacks, and sniper-fire abuse.

Dad had to negotiate decision making, social intercourse, work, and child rearing around all of this. Mum had such brief windows where she could make a rational decision. Anxiety would induce a horrible rash on her fingers. She would peel her rubber 'washing-up' gloves off and I would see the rash. At times she could not resist scratching the rash, which would of course draw blood and only make it worse. Shit! What could you do? Compassion welled up in my heart but there seemed no way to get through to her. I could only cry internally. Dad's coping mechanism was denial; pretend the nightmare was not happening. When the biggest problem was Mum's sanity, look at the ceiling, talk about the weather, do anything but acknowledge the main problem.

'Everything will be fine, son. Everything will be fine, just you wait and see.'

Brian and I would do the washing up when Mum's rash broke out and then we would be excused from the evening meal. We would get as far away as possible and put our heads in a book to gain a glimpse of what else life could offer; anything to discover a different reality.

Mum would retreat to the Bible and Dad would retreat to his shed and do things around the house, while Brian and I would independently retreat to our own rooms, rarely together. All of us isolated. I would get dragged into Mum's orbit of increased religious experiences. She managed to take us all to see the great evangelist

Billy Graham at Subiaco Oval. I had never seen so many people in one place. We were all seated on the grass and Billy Graham was up on a stage with these massive speakers booming out his message that we could all be saved. His method was first to convince us all that we needed to be saved. I didn't need a lot of convincing. I knew the Harrison family needed it badly. I couldn't take anymore so as I saw several people going forward, I got up and started to walk towards the front hearing the rapturous applause of my mother and seeing the horrified face of my father. Dad instructed Brian to go rescue me. Brian dragged me back to the family rug on the grass and I could only watch all the other lost souls as Billy Graham lay hands on their heads. They all fell backwards only to be saved from a nasty fall by the enthusiastic helpers. My redemption, the Harrison's redemption, was put on hold.

****

Mum agreed that the move to Melbourne was on and the house was sold with a sixty-day settlement. Brian was already out of there, off and married. He still had university studies to complete.

We were to catch the train the next morning for the big move east. The only trouble was that Mum had gone missing. Dad eventually tracked her down. She had escaped to Aunt Lucy's. This sad saga played out like the final act from a Shakespearean tragedy. I was reduced to a mere witness. Dad and I were standing on the grass below the front steps leading up to Aunt Lucy's porch.

'Hazel, come out and talk. I know you are there,' Dad pleaded.

There was no reaction.

'We need to talk. We are catching the train tomorrow.'

It was dead silent until we noticed two shadows pass behind the lace backing of the curtains. The fly wire door opened with a squeak and Aunt Lucy came out onto the porch.

'She doesn't want to talk to you, Milton.'

Dad pleaded again, 'Be reasonable, Lucy. Send her out. This is between Hazel and me.'

'She's too upset. She's not herself.'

'It's too late for all that. She agreed to come to Melbourne with Dennis and me.'

'She's unwell, Milton,' Lucy said.

'I know, but we can fix that,' he said none too optimistically. 'Please go in and bring her out. It can't finish like this.' When the dirty laundry is out, the dirty laundry is out. There is no more hiding. I kicked the grass with my shoe but there was a long way to go to make a big enough hole to not be there.

Aunt Lucy succumbed to the piteous request and said, 'Okay, Milton. I'll give it a go, but you stay down there you hear.'

Minutes passed, and I worked on my hole in the grass until Aunt Lucy emerged from the door supporting Mum. Mum clasped and unclasped her hands and after breaking away from Aunt Lucy's support, she rushed to the porch balustrade blurting out, 'I am not coming with you.'

'Hazel be reasonable, we've had this out together so many times. You agreed with our move to Melbourne.'

'I have changed my mind. I don't want to go now.'

'You're just having a panic attack. Once you are on the way you'll feel so much better.'

'I doubt it. I am not coming. We shouldn't have sold the house.'

'Too late. We both signed the papers.'

'You brute, you've ruined everything. I'm staying put in Perth. I am not coming,' Mum spat.

'Hazel, Dennis and I are getting on the train tomorrow morning. It leaves at nine o'clock. If you are not there then we are off without you.'

He strode to the car with great purpose, me a short distance behind. At last he had put his foot down. He had practiced appeasement and compromise all his life, but he had finally reached his limit. We retreated to Ma and Pa Harrison's house for the night. I thought it strange at the time that I was invisible to my mother. She had not pleaded for me to stay in Perth with her. She didn't even acknowledge that I was there.

PART 2 -
ADOLESCENCE
1960 – 1968

"Sometimes I know what I believe because of what I've written."

J.K. Rowling

23

CLICKETY CLACK

The *Westland* **train departed for** Kalgoorlie the next morning without Mum. Dad and I were farewelled by Ma and Pa Harrison as well as Dad's sister, Aunt Joy. There were tears and hugs all around.

We retreated to our cabin a sad twosome, mostly lost in our own thoughts trying to assimilate the happenings of the past twenty-four hours. Back then, the trip across the Nullarbor to Melbourne took a full three days. On each of those days, and several times a day, Dad would muse, 'Mum's not well but we'll be right Dennis, everything's coming up roses, son. You'll see; you could be prime minister one day.' He was trying to convince himself as much as me.

'I know, Dad' I would loyally reply. 'Jeez, I gotta say I like the menu in the dining car.' The food was a real treat.

After the turmoil of the fights and separation from Mum, we shared in the quietness with sobering personal reflection, eating in the dining car and sleeping. Dad didn't know how to share his problems with me. He took all of it on board as his problem that had nothing to do with me. So apart from the mournful 'everything's coming up roses' we didn't discuss our predicament or future. I was classified as too young for such worldly matters, and I lacked the skills to console him.

I did know though that childhood and childish things were behind me. As the train rocked from side to side advancing across each rail link 'clickety clack,' I was escaping a past childhood into a greater, albeit adolescent, period of responsibility. *Time to step up to the plate Dennis,* I told myself, *and don't let the old man down.* I was leaving Mum, my grandparents, Robbie, Uncle Ted, Daisy, Graeme, and Brian all behind. I was advancing to an unknown future.

Pa Harrison was a kindly man, an asthmatic, who was totally dominated by Ma Harrison. He gave us two books from his collection for us to read on our trip.

'You'll be needing something to read. Dennis, you'll enjoy *Robinson Crusoe* and Milton, I reckon *The Count of Monte Cristo* is a great read for you. Reading helps put into perspective your own troubles,' Pa said.

The books spoke to both of us. I know *The Count of Monte Cristo* was a favourite of my father's. Throughout his life, he would take every opportunity of watching replays of the movie and he would drag me in to share the experience. I read Patrick White's *The Tree of Man* in my late teens. All three of these books involved men being active, solving problems, and being self-reliant. The heroic men contained within the pages of these books and the concept of being manly crafted my psyche and my politics. Here was my father, in effect, a sole parent. He had no thought of government aid or other support in his predicament. He had been presented with an intractable problem and it was up to him to resolve it.

The *Transcontinental*, which ran on the Kalgoorlie to Port Augusta leg of the journey, had a fabulous observation carriage at the rear of the train. It had large windows on both sides and a curved window at the rear. There were comfortable chairs and tables liberally scattered throughout. It was a popular place to sit and read, ruminate, and doze. The train track is one of the longest straight rail lines in the world, and watching the receding track flanked by the sparse spinifex of the desert landscape was meditative. I would vacillate between thinking about everything to thinking about nothing. Dad would not always be with me. He needed his own thinking time and space, so he spent time in the cabin. He slept a lot. When he dropped off to sleep, I would sneak down to the observation car with my *Robinson Crusoe* and gaze at the retreating scenery.

I didn't really read much, it was all pretence. I thought a lot about Mum and Dad. It seemed like the end of the earth, and things would not be the same from this day forward. The world outside was flying by and although I had escaped a tumultuous household, it was the household I understood. I was polite if spoken to, but other travellers soon understood that I was a solitary sort of guy. Self-conscious about my appearance with my grey front tooth, hair brushed straight back, and developing acne I retreated into myself. I hid my grey-toothed smile behind an air of seriousness and developed a bookish persona.

Rocking in the comfort of 'clickety clack, clickety clack' with eyes closed, I reflected on my mother. Her life played out behind my eyelids. Mum was isolated in the suburbs, unable to drive a car. I think Dad couldn't trust her behind the wheel because of her mental illness. That drove her mad right into later life. Her illness isolated her further, kept her in the house. Her only real contacts were Milton, us boys, and the Martins as well as some of her wider family like Aunt Lucy. Having a mental illness was like having leprosy; people stayed away. There was a bitter relationship with Dad's family. They expressed their disappointment that he had married her, and he had ended up with this insane woman. Grandma Harrison ruled her home with an iron fist and she and Mum were hostile enemies. She was critical and unforgiving.

Unfortunately, Dad had to drive home from Perth, past Ma and Pa Harrison's Cambridge Street house in Wembley, to our home in The Boulevarde, Floreat Park. Manipulative Grandma Harrison would always dream up handyman repair jobs for Dad to perform.

'Window needs the latch repaired. Can you have a look at it?' she'd say to Dad.

'You know, Dad cannot get up the ladder anymore to clear the gutters. Could you have a go at it, son?' He didn't know how to say no and he was exploited. He was looking after two households. It drove Mum to distraction. 'You spend more time with that mother of yours than you do with me.' She would constantly accuse him of this.

'Clickety clack, clickety clack,' the record kept playing. Mum in her better days made cakes for the Methodist church cake stand but she never did charity work or really belonged to anything. Dad only half-heartedly did the Masonic Lodge thing. Life sort of stopped for them when they got married. Pre-marriage he was into rowing and cycling. She was a high society girl, spoiled and indulged in wealth. The Power's had their own tennis court and tennis parties with eligible men passing through their lives. Mum would have been a great catch for Milton as he was from a middle-class family. Ma Harrison ran a sewing business and Pa Harrison survived the Depression as a paymaster for the railways.

In Hazel's world, she would play tennis, sing, play the piano, sew, dance, paint, and work in the butcher shop learning from the sharp business brain of Pa Power. What opportunities she had missed by not capitalising on this background, I thought.

I was awakened by a hand on my shoulder, 'Dennis, we've got the six o'clock sitting for dinner.'

'Great, Dad. I wonder what's on the menu tonight.'

24

HOW HE GROW UP SO BIG THEN?

I wanted the train trip to go on forever. It was a grand escape with nothing to do but eat and think. The train journey provided the opportunity to digest food and ideas, a pattern that I have valued all my life. Above all else in life, the Descartian ability to think, to sort it out for yourself, is a quality of the highest order. The parental separation, and its resultant solitude, forced my life in a certain direction. I became less social, introverted, and searched for all sorts of information and answers in books. I understood the lack of permanence early on in life; enjoy what you have today because it could be gone tomorrow. Embrace change because there is no alternative but to do so. 'Always be grateful' is an attitude that can turn adversity into success. Be a part of the solution and not a part of the problem by assisting others when you can. I was crafted by these ideas generated by our family crisis.

I had never seen a big city such as Melbourne. The hustle and bustle of people everywhere, the smell of smoke, the bricks blackened by pollution, cars and trams, and the activity of people walking so much quicker than the Perth strollers. Where's the fire? I thought. We gathered our bags and caught two trams, the last of which was a tram down St Kilda Road to a hotel. These trams were like mini trains on their own tracks going down the centre of the road. They had their own less consistent 'clickety clack' and started with a whine as the electricity was pumped through its motors. People looked away from each other respectfully allowing some sort of privacy in the crowded confines.

The tram crossed the brown muddy creek called the Yarra River. There were cans, rotting matter, and other refuse slowly floating beneath the bridge. The Yarra was nothing like the beautiful blue of the Swan estuary, and it certainly wouldn't abound with prawns, crabs, and all the fish we used to catch there. St Kilda Road was huge with four lanes and a central road containing the tram tracks. The central road had enough room for the tram track and a car lane in either direction. The foresight that the city planners had to plan for a large city was impressive. One word, vibrancy, summed up this city. This was a city that had purpose.

St Kilda Road was lined with parklands containing mature trees and gardens visible behind them. It was a welcome softness, a green like old England, which impressed me after the dry harshness of the gum tree dominated sandy plain that was Perth.

We had arrived on a Thursday in late January. Dad had rented a house on Hawthorn Road, Caulfield in preparation of Mum and me coming to Melbourne. It was not available for our occupancy until the following Monday. I was to start school that same day at Caulfield Central School. In the meantime, Dad had organised a room in a hotel on St Kilda Road.

Dad was so assured in his movements. He already knew this city. He was a gregarious, hail-fellow-well-met sort of character, and he did his best to hide his deep underlying turmoil and sadness. The idea was to not show any weakness, to shape up and sail right, because the alternative could lead to a shipwreck. He knew the area as his ASIO office was not too distant in a grand old house in Albert Park. He seemed to know the people in the hotel and had a matey familiarity with them. He exuded a bravado that would have done Al Capone proud combined with a pretence of great wealth. On entering the hotel, it was as though his spirit had lifted, he had purpose and appeared liberated from the moroseness of the train journey. Throughout my life I observed his ability to bounce back from adversity and to not wallow in disappointment.

In the few days we had at the hotel he took me to Luna Park. Through gritted teeth, he enjoyed riding with me on the Big Dipper. Judging from his white face and stilted walk through the exit gate, it was an experience he could have done without.

When he had recovered he said, 'Let's go have a meal at Leo's, son.'

'What's Leo's?'

'It's the finest Italian restaurant you'll find anywhere in Melbourne. You haven't had Italian food, yet have you? You'll love it,' he said with a smile.

He was greeted at the door by none other than the owner, Leo himself.

'Leo.'

'Milton, you're over here again.'

'I'm here for good now. I have left Perth,' Dad replied.

'Mamma Mia! That a big move.'

'Not as far as Milano, hey?'

'No, that'a for sure,' Leo laughed.

'I would like you to meet my boy, Dennis.'

'Hello, Dennis. Welcome to the best Italian Ristorante in Melbourne,' Leo said proudly.

'Thank you, sir.'

'He has never eaten Italian before Leo.'

'No! Unbelievable! How he grow up so big then?'

'Bread and Butter pudding, I think.'

'Mamma Mia, we'll put some meat on his bones, so he can play centre half back for St Kilda. I gotta the best table in the house for you two. Comma over here near the window, and you can see the nice lady as they walka down Fitzroy Street, ha,' Leo said as he winked at Dad. I didn't quite understand why he winked at my father.

'Two spaghetti bolognaise, Leo. We have to educate the lad.'

'Uno momento, Milton.'

Two plates piled high with spaghetti and mince meat sauce arrived very quickly.

'Tuck the napkin around your neck because if you get it wrong, mince sauce gets everywhere. Now take the soup spoon there in your left hand and the fork in your right hand and copy me. You quickly twist the spaghetti around the fork while it rests on the spoon and 'voila!' There you have it,' Dad explained.

I thought this was utter sophistication and a major step up from my previous Chinese restaurant experience back in Perth. I devoured the meal and ended up with a highly decorated napkin. Leo reappeared and, as he took the plates, he said, 'For the boy, we have a tartufo on the house.'

'You are too kind, Leo. I'll have a cappuccino please while Dennis has his dessert.'

Leo brought out a chocolate ice cream ball the size of a tennis ball draped in chocolate syrup. When I broke into the ice cream there was a cherry surprise in its centre. It was delicious.

We walked away a happy, contented team. It had been a great outing, an experience to remember.

25

MORE THAN A PROJECT

Dad had selected Caulfield North Central School as it was within walking distance from the rented house just around the corner in Balaclava Road. The school was opened as Balaclava Road Primary School No 3820 two weeks before the outbreak of the First World War. In 1919, it morphed into Caulfield North Central School teaching the first two grades of secondary schooling. The school was suffering from an identity crisis as it was a halfway house between a high school and a primary school.

The Central School concept must have been driven by a crazed education bureaucracy that wanted to ease children into secondary school with some overblown protectiveness. I was shocked on the first day to find that I had to line up and march into the classroom on the tap of a kettle drum past the Australian flag. I was grateful that I did not have to salute the flag. I thought it unnecessarily nationalistic and militaristic. Memories of lining up and marching in at Floreat Park Primary flooded back to me and the stolen kisses with Daisy. This seemed so regressive after my start in the progressive Perth Modern School. Surely Dad had made a mistake when selecting this school.

The school work was unstimulating, and I seemed to be way ahead of the other students. It afforded me the time to read around the subject and explore knowledge wherever my imagination took me. I became a latch key kid with no Robbie to play with after school. I would make myself a Milo drink and have a piece of fresh bread with lashings of butter and vegemite and read anything and everything at hand after completing the desperately simple homework. There was no piano for me to play so I would put on some of Dad's records. I soon discovered the origin of Dad's 'everything is coming up roses, son.' It was from Stephen Sondheim's 'Gypsy: A Musical Fable.'

Coming home to this big, cold, dark and lifeless house sucked the life out of both of us. We dropped into a routine. I would prepare the vegetables for the main meal and when Dad arrived, he would do the cooking and then we would wash up together afterwards. There was no TV in the house so we would read books and listen to the radio and records in the lounge after dinner. Dad would put on 'The Bluebird of Happiness' and gaze into his glass of scotch. Jan Peerce's beautiful tenor voice still resonates in my ears,

"Be like I, hold your head up high,
Till you find a bluebird of happiness."

I lifted the stylus off the record player, the arm had failed to lift off. Like his life, the record was in a loop forever going round and round. Dad's head slumped forward on to his chest. I gently shook him on the shoulder.

'I'm going to bed. See you in the morning.'

'Goodnight, son. Everything's coming up roses. Another day tomorrow.' He would be asleep again before I finished brushing my teeth.

Very early on, I was required to complete an assignment for my science class. I decided I wanted to know how a car worked. Dad said, "I can help you on that project." We purchased a heavy piece of project paper, and I printed in large type "The Four Cylinder Petrol Driven Engine" boldly across the top. In our disorientated existence there were no encyclopaedias at hand, and it was well before computers and Google. Dad had no need of such things. He was a walking encyclopaedia and had an intimate understanding of the workings of car engines. Once the evening meal was over and we had cleaned up the dishes, he would say, 'Right, let's get stuck into that project.' There was no holding him back. I was staggered that he knew all this stuff. The whole workings of a car were just pulled apart and detailed into their various strategic working components and functions. The project went on for over a week and throughout the weekend. Here he was, amidst the worst time of his life, pouring everything he had into this project. He would dictate, and I would write out the details in long hand page after page. The words all flowed from him in a very structured order, and then he would pause and draw some diagrams which I would copy as neatly as possible onto the project paper. All the pages were pulled together and stapled to the top left-hand corner, and they were surrounded by all the diagrams.

We were both proud of the outcome. It was the closest I had ever been to my father and I look back on that moment with immense nostalgia. I felt he had provided unconditional love and was so heroic to do that at a time when his world had collapsed. He had given of himself so completely.

26

THE LETTER

Dad pulled me out of the Central School after eight weeks. He must have realised that it was a mistake, but more likely he was just seeking a better domestic situation. The routine of conducting his ASIO work together with cooking, cleaning, and looking after me was starting to wear him thin. He had located a place to board in Brighton. We had two bedrooms and a common sunroom in Mr and Mrs Alexander's house. They were a retired couple who required the extra income, and they were kind, considerate people. I was now attending Brighton High School and no longer coming home to an empty house. Breakfast and dinner were supplied by the Alexanders and Dad was freed up greatly.

My entry into friendship in my new school was through my sporting prowess. I played football well and became very friendly with a small firebrand boy, Percy Carmichael. I was a short, little guy but Percy was even shorter. Because of his height, he had to be smarter and tougher than anyone else. I liked him immensely. He was always jovial, quick witted, and quick footed. We both played in the same house team as rovers. Rovers in Australian Rules Football are the short fast little guys that run on the ball and pick up the crumbs (loose ball) that the big players fumble. 'Rover' is the classic all-purpose fall-back name for a dog. Playing like annoying blue heeler dogs after a juicy ankle, rovers go in where angels fear to tread and get the hard ball emerging from a pack of arms and legs disdainfully shaking off the opposition. The image of a pet dog infuriatingly out of the reach of its owner trying to recover the rag doll in its mouth comes to mind when I think of Percy.

Despite our age and because of our talent, we were selected on the school team. Also playing on the team were Carl Dietrich and Jeff Moran. Both went on to play for St Kilda. Carl had a stellar and somewhat controversial career as an athletic mobile ruckman, first with St Kilda and then with Melbourne. He was hot headed with very mobile elbows that had the habit of collecting players in the jaw and, when under threat, fast fists. He was best on the ground in his first game for St Kilda in 1963 at the age of seventeen. Naturally, as a St Kilda fan, I was there to see him play. He was exciting and brilliant. Carl was so dominant in school games that he would go up in the ruck at the centre bounce, tap the ball forward, burst through the pack at centre half forward, and kick a goal. Now this was a fine thing to witness when you were playing on the same team with him, but I had the misfortune to also play against him.

I only had the one year at Brighton High and soon moved to Elwood High to start my third year of secondary school. Again, as a junior I made the school football team. The only problem with this was that I now had to play against Carl, Jeff Moran, and my best mate Percy. Because all the Brighton boys knew me, I was a marked man and they loved to take it up to me. It was a tough grounding. I still tentatively pass my fingers over the slightly raised bone ridge behind my right ear where Carl accidently collected me with an elbow. The high C of a soprano voice brings back the memory with a harmonic resonance. The incident, however, did not stop me barracking like crazy for the rogue every time he ran out for St Kilda.

****

I still didn't have after school play mates while at Brighton, but I did like it there and was performing well academically. I achieved a third in class result for the year, and knocked around with my mate, Percy, and another bright boy Clive, who we both respected for his humour and his brains. However, towards the end of the year, I was approached by Dad.

'Do you miss your mother, Dennis?' he asked.

'I'm not sure.'

'She hasn't been well, but you know she can get better.'

'Yeah.'

'We write to each other, you know.'

'That's good, Dad.'

'I would like you to write to your mother. I would like you to tell her how much you miss her and how you would love for her to come join us in Melbourne. Do you think you could do that for me?'

I hesitated. 'Sure.'

It wasn't an easy letter to write. There were so many wounds. I didn't write it out of love for my mother, but I was motivated to do anything to stop my father's suffering.

****

Dear Mum,

I hope you are keeping well now. I am doing well at school since I moved to Brighton High. I suppose Dad told you that Caulfield Central was just not for me, all a bit strange. I have got a good friend, Percy Carmichael, and we play football together. You wouldn't believe it but he's shorter than me. They call their sandshoes 'runners,' and they have ice cream in little cardboard boxes and call them 'Dixies.' But you get used to all the new things after a while.

Dad and I are getting on well together but we both miss you terribly. I don't like seeing him so sad Mum. We love you Mum and we would really like to see you over here so that we can be a real family again. Mrs Alexander's a fairly good cook but not a patch on you, Mum. I would really like to taste your mince and sweet corn dish again, not to mention my favourite, your bread and butter pudding.

Your loving son,
Dennis.

PS: You'll love the trip on the train, and I've never seen such a good menu as the one in the dining car.

****

I showed it to Dad and he responded, 'That should do the trick, Dennis. Thank you.' I hope he could not notice that I was not as enthusiastic. I was settling into my new existence and I was nervous about more change, more drama, and more unrest.

27

LET'S START AGAIN

The Transcontinental pulled into Spencer Street station. Dad was nervously rotating his hat in his hands and winking at me as he said, 'Everything's coming up roses, eh son?'

'I hope so, Dad,' I replied. The upbeat tenor of the exchange belied our anxiety and doubts.

Mum alighted from her first-class carriage and momentarily looked lost until she spotted us. She rushed forward, and Dad and her warmly embraced. He held her tight. They kissed, no words were spoken. I could see tears in each of their eyes as they separated. Then she hugged and kissed me.

'I missed you, Dennis.'

'I missed you too.'

'I'll go get your luggage,' Dad said.

This left Mum and I together. We exchanged small talk about her journey and my schooling until she spoke.

'I am sorry, Dennis. I wasn't well when I stayed in Perth. It took me a long time to get well again. I do love you. Let's start anew, as a family.'

'Yes Mum, let's make a new start.'

With my response, she firmly pulled me towards her and held me tight. I felt that excessive possession of smothering love like drowning again. I didn't know how to respond to these feelings, but I was luckily saved by Dad's return.

Mum's life was a constant series of new starts. As I look back now, I understand her enormous courage in making all these new starts. She had to face the challenge of rebuilding relationships with her family and friends after embarrassing incidents. Dad's courage was to keep facing up, living in the hope of a better outcome, forever loyal and in love with the sweet girl that he had chosen to marry.

****

And so, I started in my fourth secondary school in two years. Dad and Mum rented a flat in Pine Avenue, Elwood, which was only a quarter of a mile to the beach and a half a mile to my new school, Elwood High School. Elwood was a lower socio-economic suburb on the shores of Port Phillip Bay, stuck between St Kilda and the prestigious Brighton. This was looking like another step back in my oscillating educational fortunes. Elwood High was a little United Nations populated by children from immigrant families. The school was eighty percent Jewish at a time when Jews formed a half of one percent of the population, but they had pooled in the St Kilda-Elwood district. There had been a 'bubble' in their emigration to Australia after both the Hungarian uprising and the overthrow of the Egyptian monarchy in 1956.

When riding my bike home from school, I never did master the three-hundred and thirty degree turn required at the junction of Glen Huntly Rd and Ormond Rd. I would arrive home with torn trousers and scrapes, scratches, and various pieces of flesh adrift. Dad, who had been a good cyclist, was convinced that I really couldn't ride. The last straw for him was when my bike, which had been a former racing bike of his, was stolen in the stairwell at the flat. The replacement bike that he bought for me reflected his lack of faith in my cycling abilities. It looked like he had collected it from the tip at no cost. It had a fixed seat that couldn't be raised or lowered; it was rusted on. It certainly didn't have gears so only direct drive was possible. The non-aligned crank arms made coordination and power distribution difficult as did the one non-rotating pedal. It only had rear brakes because some of my bigger mistakes were of my overzealous nature with the front brakes. Another common error I made was not tucking my trousers into my socks, and trouser bottoms could be caught between the chain and the teeth of the crank set.

It was a self-fulfilling judgement of my father to give me such a bike to ride. I hadn't quite cottoned on to the fact that I should maintain it myself. It was only something to get me from A to B. That same attitude transferred over to cars as I matured. I have never been a car enthusiast, nor have I ever seen them as status symbols. They have only ever been a necessary means of transport.

* * * * * * * * *

Here I was making yet another start. Who wants stability? Stability means drudgery, security, boredom. No, jump off the edge of the pier and see if you can swim. Instability and insecurity has forged my life. I do believe that growth and depth of character emerges from challenging circumstances. I fear for the strength of our present society due to the over protected upbringing of children and the developing nanny state. The attempt at normalisation and equal outcomes for all is but a futile fantasy. We bandy about concepts of diversity these days, but we try to make everyone the same instead of embracing our differences. The instability of my family and upbringing is but a mere hiccup in comparison with the stories behind each of my newfound Jewish friends. What had they endured? What had they suffered just to be sharing this schooling with me? My education was all the richer for having the opportunity to understand their plight and to befriend them.

One of the first friends I made was Chris Randall. We were both misfits, he with a severe acne problem and me with grey front tooth and minor acne. I no longer had electric shock hair. In Mum's absence, I had taken charge and now had a simple college boy style with a parting at the side. We were both good footballers and would play kick to kick after school. He was much bigger than me and played centre half forward. Every Friday we would play nine holes of golf at the Elsternwick golf course. We were very competitive. I had another one of my near miss incidents one day coming down the ninth. After eight holes, our scores were tied, so everything depended on the last hole. To increase pressure on Chris, I stood directly behind him as he played a fairway wood shot. I had miscalculated his tall stature and the length of his arms. His vigorous backswing clipped the tip of my nose and I fell back in utter surprise, tears streaming from my eyes. He won that round as I was incapable of holding a club due to my shaking. If I had stood any closer, I would have needed a full facial reconstruction or a coffin.

Basketball was a game I did not take to. I had some knock up games after school with Chris and others. Chris lived opposite the school in Glen Huntly Rd, and Mrs Randall would have me in for after school snacks with him. We would then go back onto the school grounds for basketball. I was not one of the first players picked by the two opposing captains for once. I was one of the last picked. I could not adapt to the non-contact of basketball and the difficulty of stopping the player with the ball. Football was direct with a defined way of tackling whoever had the ball. I was always fouling. My football skills did not transfer to this game.

****

Shortly after we moved into the Elwood flat, Mum found a job as a saleswoman in a dress shop in Camberwell. It meant cross suburban running around for Dad, but it became one of the best times of her life. Dad would run her to work in the morning and she would catch a series of trams to get home. She had the Power's nose for business and had always had a good eye for fashion. She had found new life. She would end a work day quite exhausted but at least she had found some happiness. I was a latchkey kid again, but happy for Mum.

The advantage of being a latchkey kid was the freedom you gained. The disadvantage was the solitude, the loneliness. Dad and I started a practice of a run along the beach in the morning, and a brief experiment of an early morning swim. I ended up with a severe bout of bronchitis and was confined to bed for a fortnight by our doctor. I didn't mind the confinement at all. I could read all the books I wanted to read instead of the prescribed school work. I learned there are advantages and disadvantages to everything in life. I have often thought that going to prison for a few years would not be exceptionally bad. It would be an opportunity to study something you were interested in and get a degree or write a book. My moralistic, Christian upbringing of course dictated that this was not an option.

Bronchial problems have plagued the male side of the Harrison family for generations. Pa was told at the age of fifty-five that he only had six months to live. He had chronic asthma, and I never saw him without an inhaler within his reach. He subsequently lived to eighty but was treated as an invalid all those years. He outlasted Ma Harrison. Brian suffered from asthma throughout his childhood and adolescent years. When we shared a bedroom at Floreat Park, my parents experimented with all sorts of different treatments. Brian would be put to bed with some inhalant concoction, wafting smoke into the air in the bed opposite from me. As I was also breathing this in it may have been acting as a prophylactic as I did not catch the Harrison weakness. Because of this recognised family weakness, Mum and Dad took my bronchitis very seriously. Dad also was forced to retire early at the age of fifty-nine. He collapsed when on an overseas posting in Athens, so he was repatriated home. The doctors suspected emphysema as he was a smoker, but ultimately the correct diagnosis was bronchial asthma. There are few things worse than seeing someone you love fighting for air. He spent the remaining fifteen years of his life fighting for air and never free from expectorating phlegm. I internally wept for him seeing him like that.

28

I HEAR YOU MASTERED HUNTINGDALE

I had been impressed with the bravado and façade my father had shown when he strode into that St Kilda hotel and when he had his interchange with Leo at the spaghetti bar. However, his ability with this trait was exceeded by his boss, Ron Richards. I referred to him as Uncle Ron. I knew him as a family friend who visited us quite regularly. He became Deputy Director of ASIO under Sir Charles Spry. I think he held a torch for Aunt Joy, Dad's sister, but I have no proof of that. He was a former London bobby who immigrated to Australia and started as a detective in the WA police force. He was a larger than life character. He looked like a living version of Dick Tracey, big chiselled face, powerful jaw, black wavy hair, and a Kevin Miller confidence that exuded charm. Never short of a word, he would put people at ease and become the focus at any gathering. He would command a room. He had mixed in high circles providing counsel to Sir Robert Menzies.

The defection of the Russian spy, Vladimir Petrov, the third secretary of the Soviet embassy in Canberra, was ASIO's greatest triumph, and through it the Australian secret service organisation gained worldwide acceptance and recognition. It was very much Ron Richards' triumph. He was the key player in all the negotiations with Petrov and took final custody of him taking him to his safe house.

Aunt Joy, at the outbreak of the Second World War in 1939, was twenty-three years old and working as a secretary to the Italian Consul in Perth. As a persona non grata, the consul fled Australia and the consulate closed. She was approached by the defence force and Commonwealth security officers to assist with the opening of the consulate safe with the thought that it may contain some secrets which could aid the war effort. She was subsequently recruited by Uncle Ron into WASS – the Western Australian Security Service. When WASS was disbanded at the close of the war in 1945, she became one of ASIO's first women employees. She was instrumental in introducing Dad to Uncle Ron which resulted in Dad's recruitment into ASIO. In its inception, the majority of ASIO was drafted from the military and Dad had worked for military intelligence in the Second World War.

****

Dad and I became St Kilda supporters, and it was a regular thing to go to the football with Uncle Ron and the Kyatt brothers who owned the famous Brighton watering hole, The Kyatt's Hotel. Uncle Ron lived in the hotel while in Melbourne. Due to his dominating personality and presence, an observer would think he owned it. We would go there and have an early lunch and then depart as a group to the football. We would arrive and always find Uncle Ron encamped at his favourite corner table consuming every morning newspaper for news, looking for some sort of edge to current affairs.

'Here's the boy that's mastered Huntingdale,' he said.

I was speechless but fittingly blushed. I had never mastered Huntingdale. I had never even played Huntingdale, a prestigious Melbourne sand belt golf course. Dad had probably told him that I regularly played the Elsternwick public course once a week with a mate, and that I could hit a good ball. I had taught myself using Tommy Armour's book 'How to Play Your Best Golf All the Time.' Later in life, I read all sorts of golf books to try and improve my game, but I wished I had stopped at this first Tommy Armour book. All the later books scrambled my brains and I never could master the game to a level that I found satisfactory.

'How are they going to go today, Dennis?'

'I am a bit worried. Verdun Howell is out and we might be a bit weak down the back.'

'You could be right young fella, but no excuses. They'll give it a good go. What will it be today for you?'

'I think I'll have fish and chips.'

'Now that is a surprise.'

'When you are on a good thing, stick to it,' I replied.

'Eh, Mortein, Dennis. Mortein.' And we both laughed.

I was the only child amongst the four men, but they never excluded me from their company. Observing their exchanges was good training in how to carry myself in personal situations. Learning the art of social discourse is so important to growing up, and I had some of the best mentors. Whether it was part of the ASIO training or the skilful recruitment, all of Dad's workmates had this air of supreme confidence and could hold the stage in all sorts of social situations. They seemed to know how to talk about any subject and still not give an iota of information away, just like a politician. Uncle Ron in full flight would place his left foot forward ahead of his right, much like a boxer, and from there the cut and thrust of verbal attacks and defence would take place. Aunt Joy was a stunningly beautiful woman. Tall, elegant, and graceful, she could vacillate between restraint and composure to laughing exuberance. As her gaiety could be relied upon, she was a favourite invitee to all the necessary espionage and/or consulate cocktail parties. She intuited the required discretion to not take a position on anything of substance and to keep the topic on trivia. She could command a room with equal ability like Uncle Ron. With her beauty and his Kevin Miller looks, if they were together at a cocktail party they would be irresistible. It is hard to imagine the two didn't have an affair, but their ASIO training meant that our family would never know the truth in this matter.

29

EQUAL DUX FORM THREE

Starting over again in a new school along with the bronchitis confinement, I had a studious, bookish year. As a result, I was equal dux of Form three with Sonya Varga.

It was in Form three that I first met another knock 'em dead beautiful Jewish girl, Michelle Frydenberg. I had many strengths but despite the excellent examples I had been surrounded with such as Dad, Uncle Ron, and Aunt Joy, verbal jousting and linguistics was not one of them. I was captain of a debate team competing against Michelle's team, and I opened my concluding argument with the words, 'I would like to attack Michelle.' Before I could get another word out, the boys in the class started rattling their desk lids and stamping the floor. They could be heard saying under their breath, 'So would we, so would we.' My face quickly reddened when I realised the construed interpreted implications of my words. Both Michelle and the teacher were not impressed. Shakily, when the furore subsided, I pushed towards a lame conclusion.

It was a hard lesson and a setback if ever I was to reach that goal of my father's 'to be prime minister one day.' I did get active within the Liberal Party in my later life, and I ran for pre-selection for both state and federal seats. Each time the members, in their wisdom, selected another candidate and I was saved from the thankless demands of a political career. My subsequent career demanded that I had a level of confidence in presentation and public speaking, so I worked hard on it by being active in Rostrum. That was a beneficial part of my overall development.

We had large class sizes at Elwood High and it is quite possible for children to bully the teacher. Any sign of weakness and a mass of rebellious children are quite capable of reducing the teacher to a quivering mess of insecurity, much like the 'Yes What?' radio series I listened to when in primary school. Once it became so out of control in our class that the teacher, whom was himself a European refugee and could not speak English well, fled the classroom holding his head in tears. The class was left in disarray and became subdued as we were left teacherless for some fifteen minutes. The headmaster then appeared and announced that Mr Brajkovic had gone home quite unwell. The headmaster was angry at the disrespectful way we had treated our teacher, and as a result the whole class without exception was held back in detention after school.

The incident left an indelible mark on my consciousness. My mother's precarious health had taught me very well just how fine the edge of the knife that separated sanity from insanity. Mob behaviour and mob rule allows no room for nicety, respect, and distinction between truth and justice, and falsehood and injustice. Mr Brajkovic had escaped a Yugoslavian hell hole to become a scapegoat to a discourteous, uncaring rabble of children playing a prank. I had received warnings from my father to avoid the peace rally turbulence of the sixties led by flower-power escapism. He told me that ASIO kept surveillance on the attendees at such rallies because, underneath it all, was the hand of the Australian communist party and international communism. Their thrust was to weaken and ultimately bring down democracies worldwide. Of course, this was decried by the progressives and left-wing moderates, but history has revealed through the regular release of cabinet papers under the thirty-year provision that this was indeed correct.

I have little respect for populist protest movements that inflame positions. There are too many willing to take up arms for causes of which they are ill informed about and intolerant of, but they persist in the belief that it is their right to disturb the activities of others. Determined to put their nose into everybody else's business they can be led by the propaganda of fear mongers. This crazy Australian trait to denounce the police, seeing them as the enemy and labelling them a 'pig,' is one that I absolutely abhor. These protestors would be the first to squeal when law and order broke down and mob rule prevailed. Our TV screens are loaded every night with the breakdown of law and order in societies throughout the Middle East and elsewhere. That is not a society I wish to live in. The intransigence of an enraged, unforgiving populace and the destruction of that society's infrastructure due to conflict saddens me greatly. Resolve differences peacefully and patiently through informed debate, not fear-emblazoned ideology.

30

INSPIRED BY MR WILL

I **felt the tug between** wanting to belong and be accepted, and being independent, my own person, an individual above the crowd. The turbulence of my continual school switches and the insecurity of my family situation pulled me towards an isolationist approach to life. It would have been easy to adopt the 'outsider' persona but my sporting ability tied me to society and people. In my first year at Elwood High, I was elected captain of the under fifteen Saturday morning football side and I went on to receive the best and fairest player award for the season. This achievement shunted me into the first eighteen the following year, and I wasn't even yet in the senior grades. It was a continuation of the pattern of playing sports above my age group. I went down as a junior to the Elsternwick Sub District cricket club and played with their juniors. Once when they were short a player I was promoted to the second eleven. I was on a hat trick, bowling the leggies that Uncle Ted had taught me. Dad's chest was so pumped up clapping with excitement that he nearly fell head first over the fence.

I did go on to get a hat trick in schoolboy cricket in front of my hero, Mr Will. The third wicket was obtained against a batsman that had little talent, and I had a ring of players in position for a catch. The batsman obliged and hit a ball he could undoubtedly have left alone but like a bee to a honey pot, he had to have a go. Sometimes there is just too much time to think when facing a slow bowler, and in some drugged mesmeric state the batsman attempted to hit the ball. As the ball was caught, I was in utter surprise and jubilant. Mr Will thought it amazing and shared in the moment presenting me with the ball. I had experienced yet another moment of sporting success and exhilaration.

****

Mr Will was the senior maths master at the school. I looked up to him, and he was the most influential of all my teachers. He would stride into the classroom with great purpose bedecked in academic robes and, in the case of special ceremonies, added the mortar board complete with tassel. He wore these with great pride, and he exuded style. He had my complete respect and taught more than just mathematics. He talked philosophy, expounded ideas, and he challenged us to be bigger entities in our world and explained ideals that were worth defending. I added him to my list of people that I did not wish to let down. I wanted to do my best for him, to succeed. He reinforced my ability to think, and to admire the beauty contained in high level thought. He increased the difficulty of the mathematical puzzles that we had to unlock and explained a complete logic and thought process that, if followed, provided full proof.

Because of his teaching I wanted to become a mathematician. I loved the honesty, the truth, the splendour, and the logic that powered mathematics. I loved the fact you could play by the rules and know when you were either right or wrong. Quad errat demonstrandum means "what I have set out to do I have demonstrated," signalling the proof of a mathematical theorem. It represented all I wanted to know or pursue in life. If you could just be one of the most brilliant minds, it would be possible to live some erudite, academic life in an unchallenged, protective cocoon. What other pursuits provide the utmost certainty that you are right? The knowledge that you had the correct answer was so empowering, I found it intoxicating. In the end, the pursuit was not to merely get the correct answer but to achieve it in the most efficient and elegant manner.

It took me to the middle of my second year at Melbourne University when I was finally broken from the dream. The Pure Maths II class was being addressed by a lecturer scribbling unintelligible symbols on the blackboard. Encumbered with long, ill-kept hair he was dressed in shorts with long, wool, knee-length socks that were inserted into sandals, for this was the depths of a

Melbourne winter. To add to the ignominy of the presentation he did not really address the students, but all we saw was his back as he talked to the blackboard. Was he really trying to give us information here? Is his passion for the topic supposed to magically cross the ether to inspire students? Is this the mentor to which I wish to emulate for my future? I think not. My juvenile, altruistic bubble had burst. I had reached a place whereby I could not understand one thing this man was attempting to teach. It was then I switched to my new passion, geology.

31

THE RICHMOND METHODISTS

My father constantly encouraged me, 'You could be prime minister one day, son. You're a leader of men.' Whilst young and with thoughts of invincibility, there is a tendency to believe the rhetoric that flows your way. There is no doubt that encouragement enables, and the converse is equally true, discouragement disables. My entry into Elwood High had been dramatic with both immediate academic and sporting success. It had gained me several friendships.

Flush with my football success, I worked out how to catch the tram to St Kilda to train with the under sixteen St Kilda fourths. I was the first of any Elwood High student to have done so, so in that sense, Dad's voice echoed in my head, 'You're a leader of men.' And several others followed, first amongst them being my friend, Chris, but also the two Rays and the two Garys. We were required to train on both Tuesday and Thursday nights. I had two seasons with them playing variously as a rover, a wingman or half forward flanker. I was promoted once to sit on the bench as a reserve for the under eighteen thirds. I sat there all day in my dressing gown and they never let me run on. It was such a disappointment and I was denied the bragging rights to tell my grandchildren that I had played for St Kilda thirds. My story would have to remain for eternity, 'I played with St Kilda fourths.'

****

To a fifteen-year-old, all grown men look old. Our coach looked old, he was short, rotund, and out of shape. I thought it was maybe a snapshot of my future. This could be what happens to rovers as they age. One clever trick too many and you come out of a pack with a smashed-up face and a wonky knee preventing you maintaining your fitness. He'd earned his stripes and I respected him, always trying to implement his instructions. I particularly remember the occasion when he had a one-on-one with me one day during half time. We were playing at the MCG against Melbourne and I was on the wing getting a bath. I couldn't get near the ball.

'You're getting done over, Dennis,' he said.

'Yeah, I know coach. Not my day.'

"Listen, why don't you rough him up a bit?'

'How?' I asked.

'Just give him a niggle or two. You know, elbow in the ribs, tap his ankle with your boot, all that light stuff. See how he reacts.'

'I'll give it a go.'

'Good boy, Dennis.'

Junior football at the MCG attracts only a small crowd and they all gather around at the wings. So, when I started my mobile elbow and foot tapping antics they were all too visible to the gathered spectators. I quickly became the number one enemy, and there were plenty of words given to the umpire about my unsporting play. Dad didn't claim me and silently receded to the back of the gathering. I was robotically carrying out my instructions and suddenly, I was getting the ball and lots of free kicks. I had enraged my opponent so all he cared about doing now was to knock my block off. The tables had turned, and I had a great second half of football.

The coach proudly threw his arm on my shoulder after the game and said, 'Great game, Dennis! That's another trick to put in the cupboard and bring out when you need it. You helped turn the game round.'

I was a stayer, not a sprinter, and at my best when on wet grounds which slowed the fast players up. As I had the stamina I was also at my best in the last half as the others tired. In addition, I had to be crafty and I developed some illegal ways of getting free kicks. A particular favourite of mine was grabbing an opponent's arm and drag it over my shoulder when flying for a mark, knowing that the umpire was unsighted. That was a highly productive method of getting an around the neck free kick. Other favourites were tapping the ball away from a player as it fell between his hand to foot as he was attempting to kick it and the opponent would have an airy. And it was extraordinarily satisfying to time a bump to the side such that the opponent didn't have a leg to stand on. That is, his nearside leg was in the air and he was only standing on his far leg.

****

At the following Thursday night practice, after the Melbourne match, the coach called us together near the boundary line under the lights.

'Look boys, I know you have all heard the rumours and stories about the Richmond Methodists. Their coach has given me his cast iron guarantee. There will be no trouble on Saturday. They've turned over a new leaf and will just be playing football.'

We were gathered in a circle with light rain falling. I looked around the circle of my teammates and I saw something more than light reflect back from their eyes. I saw fear. We had heard things through the grapevine about the Richmond Methodists. They were coached by 'Slugger' Nelson who ran a boxing studio down Bridge Road, Richmond. Football was secondary to their boxing bouts and undertaken by Slugger as part of their fitness regime. They had been in several brawls with other sides.

'Not only have I spoken to Slugger but I have had a word to Reverend Jones as well. He told me the boys will be on their best behaviour.'

I looked around the circle again and I could sense a degree of disbelief towards the words we were hearing. I had double doubts because I knew from the coach's previous lesson last week at the MCG that it was quite easy for a coach's attitude to seep through to the players at the drop of a hat. What if Slugger gave his players some instructions like I had received?

'The van's leaving right at seven thirty. See you then boys.'

We were transported to each of our games as a group in a large 'Gronow' furniture van. It was designed to unite us as a football team. Hanging on to straps suspended from the sides of the van, we travelled to the Burnley oval which was situated right alongside the Yarra. The mist had not lifted, and thick dew was atop the ground. We had hoped the mist would lift by eight thirty when the game would start. Our coach led us into the changing rooms and said hello to Reverend Jones as he passed.

'Nice day for football Reverend,' our coach said.

'God's own, God's own.'

On a big whiteboard the coach scrubbed out a couple of names and moved players around. Once in our football gear he told us to have a look at the board. Not too many surprises. Chris was still at centre half forward. I liked to look out for my mate, Chris. Big Barry of course was in the ruck with Ray, and Larry and I were the rovers for the day, changing in the forward pocket.

'Now all you have to do is play football boys. There will be no trouble. Reverend Jones tells me that they are just a bunch of angels.' There was dead silence.

'Joke boys. It was a joke.'

'Do you think they'll know I'm Jewish?' Serge asked.

'Don't be daft, Serge. Of course, they won't unless you tell them.'

'Okay that's alright then.'

'Coach, I was a Methodist once,' I spat out.

'They won't be worried about that, Dennis. Now, I wouldn't provoke them if I was you. None of those tactics I told you to use last week, alright?'

'Of course. Understood coach.'

With that, we ran out on the ground pumped up and ready for the contest in the lion's den, although it should be the tiger's den as Richmond's nickname was the Tigers.

When I was resting in the forward pocket, the tattooed specimen of developing manhood that was my opponent was telling me about the fight he had at Festival Hall the night before. 'Yeah, I bashed his lights out in the fifth. It was great.' He emphasised the point by smiling his toothless smile at me while punching a fist into his other stationary hand.

The impact made a loud disturbing sound and I meekly said, 'Good for you.'

We came in at half time and the score line was St Kilda ten goals one point to Richmond Methodists no score.

As we sucked on our oranges the coach walked around and gave us encouragement, repeating, 'I told you everything was going to be alright. All you have to do is play football and keep out of any fights.'

After half time I opened on the ball and soon received a punch behind the ear. I called Larry in and retreated to the forward pocket. It happened quickly, and I didn't know where it came from. As I was resting I noticed Ray receive a blow in the centre of the ground after he had kicked the ball. Ray reacted and that was the sign for the Richmond Methodists. Players raced to the centre of the ground where there was an all-in donnybrook. Punches and kicks were thrown freely, even the umpire was attacked. The umpire declared the game to be over. Parents and officials directed us towards the change rooms. The ineffectual Reverend Jones was saying, 'Now, now boys, stop this rowdy behaviour. You said you would be good today.' Several mothers had elevated umbrellas to beat the Richmond Methodists off our backs.

Somehow, they shepherded us all into the change rooms and the police and the 'Gronow' van was called. The Richmond Methodists were blood crazy and followed us to the rooms and thumped on the door, yelling, 'Come out and fight you buggers, come out and fight.'

When the police arrived, like the Holy Ghost, none of the Richmond Methodists remained or there may well have been some arrests. We were escorted to the van and departed. I massaged the lump behind my ear. It had been applied above the Carl Dietrich lump. But I had gotten off lightly, Ray's nose was spread all over his face and Big Barry's also looked askew. Chris was covered in blood and the inside of the van was like a large ambulance. It was decided to run the van to the hospital and have us all checked out.

'They'll be rubbed out of the competition for this,' our coach kept repeating.

The following week it finally came to pass, they were banned. You would have thought that was the end of it until the press became involved a week later and a journalist fabricated false pity for the Richmond Methodists, claiming that all they wanted to do was play football. Haydn Bunton Jnr, a renowned football star of an earlier era, was passing through Melbourne and conned into making a similar statement. Sensational and 'causal' journalism with much the same distorted standards are constantly with us.

32

DRAMA AT THE PALAIS THEATRE

I did have an element of the devil in me back then, a mischievous spirit which would get me into trouble. I recall being very disruptive in music classes. Music was a compulsory class which involved singing en masse and recorder playing. With classes of thirty-six or more, it was chaotic for the teacher and they were easy prey for students out for a good time. As a non-core unit, marks in music were meaningless, so whole groups of us would act dumb, singing deliberately off key and at the top of our voices. There was little the teacher could do. She probably thought we were a particularly unmusical sample of the general population. As I look back on it now I realise it was an educational opportunity forever lost due to my immaturity. Wisdom comes but slowly.

In addition, respect and reputation is earned over a history of incidents and experiences. I had been selected as a likely candidate for prefect in the following year due to my high academic and sporting achievements as well as my popularity with fellow students. This unravelled on a school excursion to the ballet at the Palais Theatre in St Kilda which is located alongside Luna Park.

I still did not understand girls. I was much more comfortable with girls out of my life than in it. I was being pursued by Geraldine McPhee. She was putting out all the signals that she wanted me to be her boyfriend, but I had no idea how to play this game. She was attractive but not so stunningly beautiful that my heart missed a beat. She did have very well kept beautiful, shoulder length mousy hair that bounced as she walked. In fact, all of her bounced as she walked. She had a small nose that was strangely pinched in at the base of the nostrils accompanied by numerous freckles on her face. She was inseparable from her friend Carol Broad.

It was all very flattering being hunted, but I did not know where to take such advances. I do recall Geraldine and Carol bouncing up and down barracking at an interschool football match and I put in an extra effort to win the ball next to the boundary line right alongside them. Male gallantry to win the heart of the maiden? Due to their close proximity, I experienced momentary animal lust.

They manoeuvred me into inviting them to the pictures. It was 'them.' They were inseparable and well trained as there was safety in numbers. They selected the movie, 'Pepe.' I couldn't understand the movie at all, but that was because I couldn't think. Geraldine held my hand and that smothering, captured feeling of entrapment swept through me. I didn't know then that Carol was suppressing her own feelings towards me but didn't express them, preferring to leave me to Geraldine's manipulation. Sweat broke out on my forehead and transferred to my hands. Such closeness to a girl was nerve-racking. I was not ready for this experience. I felt threatened. I was not prepared to give myself to another or be so possessed. I couldn't get out of there quick enough. We caught our separate trams home after the pictures and I swore never to get myself in such a pickle ever again.

Our next outing together was the school excursion to the ballet, but thankfully it wouldn't be cool to sit alongside them. The supervising teachers made sure that the boys were separated from the girls. A few sly, stolen glances were exchanged as we entered the bus.

Dame Margot Fonteyn and Rudolph Nureyev stopped mid-pirouette and walked smartly off the stage. The music in the orchestra pit faded out and the theatre lights went on. This was most unusual, they are professionals and surely the show must go on. An announcement came over the PA system and dramatically filled the hall: 'The principal dancers will not continue the pas de deaux unless the school children are brought to order and there is complete silence throughout the performance. Teachers, bring your pupils into order and I will negotiate with Dame Margot and Rudolph.'

Miss Rowan, the Deputy Head Mistress, rose to her full height which was five foot with the assistance of her matronly solid high heels and her raised coiffured hair. With narrow, steely eyes she surveyed the rows of Elwood High School students under her tutelage. These students were meant to be ambassadors for the school, how dare they put its reputation at risk. Elwood was not the only school attending this special matinee performance by Fonteyn and Nureyev, but Miss Rowan was convinced that this was a problem caused by an Elwood pupil. At about the same time I thought, Ma'am, it wasn't me.

There was an explosion of colour on Miss Rowan's face. It started just as a pink alteration around her neck but then travelled to a brighter red throughout her face. At that moment I could not distinguish her lips from her skin, and then her nose became scarlet. This was not looking good. My antennae rose but not quick enough. She was scanning the students for a scapegoat.

I had received a lot of good advice from my father over the years, most of which seemed to make sense, and I didn't question it very closely. One such advice was, 'Always look people in the eyes, son.' Well yes, good advice, but as I looked Miss Rowan in the eye I, ever in the moment, must have had a remnant smile on my lips.

'You! Yes you, Dennis! You come here. I know you are the ringleader of this outlandish behaviour. You are going to sit alongside me for the rest of the concert, and I don't want to hear another word out of you. You and me will be visiting the headmaster when we return.'

'Probably not an appropriate time to point out to Miss Rowan that it should be "you and I," I thought. 'Is that a hue of purple on the tip of her ear?' I just had to be the fall guy. Under these circumstances, mere words and negotiation would just not be possible. The only advantage of this humiliation was that it placed me amongst the girls. Taking my seat alongside Miss Rowan, I looked down the row and there was the stunning Michelle Frydenberg, all prim, proper, and pert. Miss Rowan soon realised where my eyes were roaming, and she put her elbows out like a pair of wings and pinned me to the back of my seat. 'Oh hell, the inequity of being a victim,' I thought.

'Nothing for it but to watch the ballet.' The incident was to have a far-reaching effect on me – that's the end of being elected a prefect next year. Miss Rowan and the Senior Master would have casting votes and she would also hold great sway with the other teachers.

Oh my God, it was hard to breathe. This petite woman had a presence beyond her physical frame. Here come Dame Margot and Rudolph Nureyev back on stage, the one with dainty little steps, the other with that funny walk as though there was chewing gum stuck to the bottom of his shoes.

I couldn't understand this art form at all. It seemed to be all about, 'Look at me, look at me! Run here, run there! Have another look at me!' It was all about the woman. The man seemed to be just a prop around which the woman moved. No wonder women love it – they are dominant, king pin, or rather queen bee – the man a mere servile entity, there to be a tool used for physical stunts.

Dame Margot twirls around Nureyev a few more times. I couldn't even go to sleep as steel-eyed Miss Rowan would not cease with the lateral scans going left and right – there was to be no more disturbances from Elwood High. This whole art form seemed to be so frustrating. The woman teases and flirts with the man, so titillating. How much more can a man take? No wonder women love it; it is the longest form of foreplay so far designed on the planet.

The performance ended to polite applause and lots of bowing, more clapping and more bowing and we were hustled off to the bus transport back to school. On board, Michelle Frydenberg asked, 'Oh, wasn't that just beautiful, Dennis?'

'Oh, yes,' I replied. 'I didn't see much of Nureyev though. Tell Geraldine and Carol I had nothing to do with the commotion, will you?'

'Yes, of course,' responded Michelle with an audible sigh, 'because we all know how reliable you can be.'

This wasn't to be my last failure, in the eyes of women that is, when it comes to ballet. Several years later, I was with my wife, Kathy, at a performance of Swan Lake by the Australian Ballet at the Sydney Opera House. Wave after wave of ballerinas in tutus advanced towards me, gliding left then gliding right. My God, it was good for a while but then fatigue overcame me, and I started the uncontrollable head nod. Embarrassed, Kathy nudged and prodded me throughout the performance. It took months to get out of the doghouse for that one.

Many years later, I was seated with Kathy in our family room watching the Australian Ballet's golden anniversary gala concert. Slowly, I leaned forward and adjusted myself into the alert position. Ballet is a very advanced art form. There is no voice, only movement and music to tell the story. Something for the new age 21st century Millennial to learn from. It is necessary to concentrate and be totally absorbed in the moment; multitasking is impossible. Ballet can say things in a form that no other medium, perhaps apart from poetry, can. It's much like sculpture in the making, forever changing until the final act – feel the dancer's chisel as they extract from the void some invisible and unfathomable cosmic truth.

Maturity for a man is not going to sleep at the ballet but understanding and enjoying it. It had taken me fifty years of growth to reach that level of maturity. Michelle Frydenberg was in that same space when she was sweet sixteen. John Gray showed great insight when, in1992, he wrote *Men Are From Mars, Women Are From Venus.*

Still, give me credit; it's a journey that many men have not yet completed.

33

SCHOOL MILE TRIUMPH

In Form five, with my prefect ambitions thwarted, I was happy to take second prize and was elected captain of one of the Sporting Houses. By now I was becoming aware that my father's forecast of becoming prime minister one day could be a difficult assignment. I knew I had been blessed with many gifts, but I was now appreciating the diverse gifts of others, their writing abilities, their political and social conscience, their understanding of history and much more. My developing awareness of the depths of the human experience and the variety of talents prompted me to examine the pursuit of sporting versus academic excellence.

The pursuit of knowledge won out in the end, but I still had one or two pieces of sporting glory left to experience. I won the school mile in my final two years at school and the eight-hundred and eighty yards race in my final year as well. The first win was the most memorable. The sporting carnival was held at Olympic Park. I was gone for all money and, at the two-hundred and twenty-yard mark from the finish line, I looked ahead to Robert de Kleyne who was already half way down the straight to the finish. I decided to give it a go and, rising on my toes, I started sprinting to run him down. Robert de Kleyne was a six former and school champion swimmer. It did not seem right that he should also be an athletics champion. This thought spurred me on as well as the knowledge that Dad was at the event, keenly watching. He liked taking stories back to Uncle Ron, his work colleagues, and the Kyatts, our St Kilda supporter friends, to brag about how well I was doing.

Robert de Kleyne didn't know I was coming until it was too late for him and he couldn't kick start himself again. I passed him in the final dash for the line. The victory won me great acclaim, with a large photo on the back page of the Age the following morning, but it was of greater pleasure to perform so well before Dad, Mr Will, and yes, Geraldine, Carol, and Michelle. The experience taught me the invaluable lesson of never giving up despite the odds or the predicament. There is such a fine line between victory and defeat.

34

MY ADOLESCENT MATES

Everyone needs people in their lives who are genuine mates. In Fourth form I discovered Dave Slipper and Trevor Wakefield. We became firm friends. Trevor and I would drift around to Dave's place after school and talk and muck around. Up until these two friends, my life had been one competition or another either with schoolwork or sporting endeavours.

Dave's place became the focus because Trevor's dad was an in-and-out of work alcoholic, and my existence living in the cramped confines of a flat provided no opportunity for free expression. Dave's place had a great backyard, a house that breathed space, and his parents were tolerant, non-judgemental, and likeable. They seemed indifferent to his immediate success and gave him space and time to develop. The freedom afforded to him by his parents was a revelation to me. Mr Slipper was a house painter and as he worked tradesman hours, I saw a little bit of him. He was a jovial, happy character and upon arriving home from work he would always have a welcoming chat with Trevor and me.

Dave had accepted different challenges in his life, *Boys Own* type challenges. He seemed to know who he was early on in life. There was no confusion and he exuded a *Hemingway* manliness, a confidence and bravado akin to Uncle Ron, but he was only a teenager. He was different and had different dreams. He had no sporting or academic achievements to look back on like Trevor and I, but we were the followers and Dave was the leader. Life had become serious for Trevor and me because of our different family situations, but Dave being from a happy family was becoming his own man.

He showed me a different form of courage, not the manufactured courage of facing a fast bowler or going into a pack to get the ball at football. All of that had become second nature to me due to my technique lessons from Uncle Ted and years of practice. No, the real courage is accepting new challenges, outside your expertise, putting in for your mates and always supporting each other. Mixing with Dave was giving me a window into a different life.

His interests were with motor sports, both bikes and cars, archery, guns, hunting, fishing, and camping. Trevor and I were still trying to sort out girls but Dave didn't have much interest in them; they were peripheral to his existence. Some of the things he would dream up seemed outlandish and developed on a whim.

'I've got no work on Sunday. Let's hitchhike to Frankston, bum around, have lunch, and hitchhike home,' Dave said.

Trevor and I would have a hundred practical reasons why this wasn't such a good idea, but we rarely aired them; we didn't want Dave to see us as wimps. Sometimes we would try and outdo each other and be the first to say, 'Great idea, let's do it.' That would put heavy pressure on the last to commit.

Trevor and I always seemed to be botting off Dave. He had money because after school and on weekend rosters he worked down at Des Casey's Ampol service station. At five shillings an hour accumulating wealth was a slow process, but Dave was on the way. He had been working for a year or two by now. He respected and believed in himself. He would always purchase first class gear. In contrast, Trevor and I shopped at the Op shop end of town.

He had the best weightlifting gear as he was always working on his fitness and body image. This was all new to me. I had been warned by my father for years not to get into weights. 'Bad for you, son. Once you stop you run to fat,' Dad would say. So, I gave it no more thought. Mind you, Dad had made a few bad calls as my personal trainer. He insisted in feeding me steak and eggs before my Saturday morning games with St Kilda. I would run onto the field with a heavily distended stomach. Maybe that's why I finished a match well because it wasn't until the last quarter that energy could transfer from my stomach to my legs.

'You fellows are always broke. You've got no money. Why don't I introduce you to Des Casey? He needs more guys serving petrol.'

'I'm in,' Trevor said.

What could I do? I was the last to respond, 'Great idea, me too.'

Dave and Trevor were to become my best man and groomsman respectively. Dave left school after his Leaving Certificate while Trevor and I matriculated and went on to university. Naturally, he had more money than either of us as we slogged on with our education. As a result, he led the way in most things, especially in getting a first car.

35

A WEE BIT OF ROAD RAGE

No sooner had I established these new friends than we were upping stumps once more. Mum and Dad had tired of the flat and at the end of my second year at Elwood High bought a house in Glen Iris, ten kilometres away as the crow flies, or fifteen kilometres across the orthogonal Melbourne road grid. It was decided that I could finish my secondary schooling at Elwood. It would have been much easier to go to Camberwell High, but I was so well established at Elwood. It meant however a lot of travel. Dad would drive me to school each morning and I would catch two trams home crossing a multitude of suburbs. The drive to school could be exciting at times, going along the roads that were shared between cars and trams.

I saw the best and worst of my father during these delivery runs to school. It automatically gave us time together and he would plug into my schooling progress and encourage me no end to advance towards being prime minister one day, although by now he really should have understood that I had a scientific bent. Unfortunately, when he was under pressure I did see some deplorable road rage incidents. One time he had stalled the car at the lights and, in trying to start it again, flooded the carburettor. I knew this because of that fabulous project we had done together while renting at Caulfield. I wisely refrained from advising him that was the problem. The driver behind us was aggressively blowing his horn. Dad got out of the car and walked up to the horn blower and said, 'Listen mate, you get my car started and I'll blow the horn for you.' I thought this was one of his finest hours.

One of his not so great hours though was when he took offence at a driver cutting in on him. He and the other driver were valiantly trying to pass on the inside of a tram as we all raced down High St Malvern; not an easy task in peak hour traffic with closely spaced tram stops. The offender was now one car ahead of us and Dad wanted to get even, so a protracted game of cat and mouse commenced whereby he would race up behind the tram looking for an opening to dart in front of this rotten citizen travelling on our inside. Not a word was said, and I braced myself in the front passenger seat with increasing tension in my legs, heart pounding. I thought I was merely going to school but instead I was thrust into a bitter contest. This must be the excitement Dave spoke about with motor racing; for me it was just plain frightening.

Dad saw his opening and went for it. I was thrust back in my seat as he gunned it. The opening, however, had closed because the other driver had floored it at the same time. Any collision is very noisy, this one particularly so as rotten citizen's front bumper was stripped clean off. Like the last yards on the big dipper ride at Lunar Park the two cars came to a slow halt on the side of the road. The tram now long in the distance, Dad said, 'You stay in the car, Dennis. I'll deal with this jerk.'

It wasn't easy as I had to swivel right around but I took quick, furtive glances at the pair as they exchanged heated words, among the essential contact details. I managed to quickly have eyes forward when Dad returned.

'Well, that's that. There are some mugs in this world,' he said.

'Yeah, bloody bad luck.'

Nothing else was said for the rest of the trip. When he dropped me off I said, 'Have a good day, Dad.'

He quietly mumbled, 'Thanks mate and you.'

I wasn't on my game that day at school being all fidgety and massaging my neck, mathematical problems seemed obtuse and unsolvable.

'What's wrong with you today, Dennis?'

'Late night, Mr Will. Just a bit sleepy.'

36

EXCURSIONS INTO SCIENCE

The move to Glen Iris placed Mum closer to her work in the dress shop in Camberwell. It may well have been the primary motivation for the move, but I was not part of the decision. I learned to adapt. I introduced myself to a new group, the Camberwell Sub District Cricket Club. I started with the fourth eleven and again threw myself into my studies.

Down the backyard of the house was a shed with a low ceiling that had been built onto the side of the garage, probably as a garden shed. It was assigned to me and it served as my study for the next five years as I completed both my secondary and tertiary studies. Stripped of the opportunity I experienced in the previous year to muck around with Dave and Trevor after school, I became solitary once again. The study doubled as both a laboratory and experimental workshop. I started with a basic chemistry set but then expanded out buying chemicals from supply shops. I had a chart of the periodic table on the wall and conducted all sorts of experiments. I always found chemistry interesting and absorbing, so I immersed myself in it. I didn't merely do chemistry homework, I expanded upon it and went to the next level of hands-on understanding.

My scientific curiosity then moved to electronics. I would buy the latest radio electronics magazines, and try and understand electrical circuits, their component parts, capacitors, resistors, batteries, and switches. I found it fantastically interesting and challenging, but I intuitively knew I was only picking up a small fraction of what it was all about. Physics is a more demanding discipline than chemistry to master. My electronics brilliance peaked when I made a crystal set. The crystal set only ever tuned in to one station, 3AW, and I was very fortunate to even get that as it had only come to air one week prior to the end of the project. In winding my tuning coil, I think I had put too many loops on it, therefore limiting its tuning capacity. I never did solve that problem as my mind had moved on to other challenges.

Despite these excursions into practical science, mathematics remained my one true love. I matriculated with a Commonwealth Scholarship with second class honours in physics and chemistry, and only a pass in my two mathematics subjects. That was a disappointment and a mystery to me as I had devoted myself wholeheartedly to maths above all else. At university, the only honours I received was in first year chemistry, and I have already related that Pure Maths II saw me peak out in my beloved subject.

37

WHITE BOOTS

It was in my last year of school that I fell in love with Barbara Redding. I hadn't progressed very far in the love stakes. I was still being pursued by Geraldine McPhee and Carol Broad, though why I don't know as I had given them little encouragement. I was still getting over the claustrophobia of holding hands during the 'Pepe' movie. Girls had remained a distant third to sports and education. I attended a co-ed school, so I knew they were there, but I had no concept of how you were supposed to interact with them. It all seemed too hard, too much bother. It was much easier to go kick a football or muck around with the fellas. Then something changed, and I began to realise that they may be interesting after all.

I was drawn towards this striking girl, at least to my inexpert eyes anyways; Barbara. She was quite aloof and a challenge. The tables had been turned; instead of being chased, I was doing the chasing. She was a British girl, very reserved and refined in her speech. I had no concept of how blokes impress and win over girls. Maybe it was not important enough to me yet. We had had the odd malted milk together down at the deli and held hands as I walked her to her tram. She lived in the adjacent suburb, Caulfield; a much more salubrious suburb than Elwood. It was approaching the end-of-year school break up and the Christmas holidays. Naturally, I moved to thoughts of an appropriate Christmas present for my first ever girlfriend.

I had never been that good or imaginative in selecting Christmas presents. My mother had run out of cupboard space for the pepper and salt shakers I had bought her over the years. I thought it'd be better that I buy Barbara something other than pepper and salt shakers. So, I soon noticed these fabulous white boots in a shoe shop.

They were bright, glossy leather with a zip up the side, and they went all the way to just under the knees. I thought, 'Gees, wouldn't Barbara look fabulous in those with navy blue jeans tucked into the top.'

Of course, the next problem was how to afford them. They weren't cheap – forty pounds. Still, I had been solving maths problems all year. 'What's another problem?' I asked myself. I could scrape together twenty pounds, but where to get the remaining twenty pounds from? I wasn't going to approach my parents because then they would know about Barbara. I wasn't ready for that kind of scrutiny. The only possibility would be Dave and Trevor. Surely, they would help a man in distress?

****

We three were doing part time work at Des Casey's as grease monkeys and tarmac attendants. Back in the 60's, the competitive edge in business was to provide service, a novel concept not often employed in today's cost-cutting, just-in-time management. As the cars rolled in we would serve the customers, greeting them with:

'And how much would you like today, Sir or Madam?'

'Can I check your oil, water, tyres?'

'Would you like your windscreen cleaned?'

It paid five shillings an hour. So, with four hours of work you could earn twenty shillings or one pound. Australia back then had forty-hour work weeks so ten pounds represented a week's work for us. To this day I cannot remember the persuasive words I used on Dave and Trevor to get them to part with ten pounds each of hard-earned money. I didn't have the gift of the gab back then. Maybe it was out of pity for a love-struck adolescent. It was most likely their first glimpse of such a person, but it wouldn't be their last. That's what friends are for, I guess.

****

I had never been to Barbara's house in Caulfield before. It involved a long walk and a tram ride to get there, but I thought it would be well worth it to see her and surprise her with my Christmas present.

It was a grand house with beautifully manicured shrubs and flowers in the garden. I noticed a red Triumph TR3 parked in the drive way. 'Wow, what a car. Must be her brother's,' I thought. I entered the front gate which squeaked iron upon iron. This imperfection strangely made me feel more at home as I strode to the door to ring the bell.

The door was opened by an older version of Barbara, and I asked, 'Hello Mrs Redding, I'm Dennis. Is Barbara home?'

'Oh, yes,' she replied. While turning, she cried, 'Barbara! You have a visitor.'

Barbara appeared at the door her eye lashes blinking demurely.

'Dennis, what a surprise to see you,' she said as she pulled the front door closed behind her.

'Barbara, I have a little Christmas present for you.'

'Oh, you shouldn't have.'

And with that I gave her the large decorated box with a Christmas card attached. She opened it and was rendered speechless at the sight of the boots.

'I hope you like them. If they are not the right size you can take them back, but I think you'll find they are okay. I took a print of your runners when you were not looking.'

She recovered enough to kiss me on the cheek and said, 'These are just beautiful, Dennis. I will treasure them forever.'

I managed to kiss her back on the cheek and said, 'Have a nice Christmas.'

She responded, 'Yes, Happy Christmas to you too.' I then turned and left giving a little perfunctory wave from the front gate.

Somehow, I felt a little hollow and empty in the pit of my stomach. I had got something wrong here. It didn't seem much return for my gift.

****

They pulled in to the service station in the TR3 with the motor vibrating vigorously beneath the long, red bonnet – all energy, hard to contain, urgent for action.

Dave looked at me and said, 'That's yours mate.'

'You bastard,' I responded.

'Nice motor, sir. How much would you like today?'

'Fill her up.'

'Right you are. And can I check your oil, water, tyres, sir?'

'Yes, thanks. And clean the windscreen if you would.'

I finished with the petrol, oil, water, and tyres, and as he left to pay the bill I started on the windscreen.

'Hello Barbara, nice to see you,' I said to her as I cleaned the windscreen and looked down upon her.

'Lovely to see you too, Dennis.'

'See you've got the boots on.'

'Yes, I love them. Thanks awfully,' she said as she fluffed her hair up.

'Just out for a spin with your brother?'

'Yeah.'

****

'Barbara's just out for a spin with her elder brother,' I remarked to Dave as I wiped my oily hands on an old rag.

'Sure, and Sophia Loren is my aunt. You're so naïve, man.'

'Beats being a suspicious prick,' I snapped back.

'Believe what you like. You're simple man.'

'How much do I owe you?'

'Six quid – just another twelve hours work. Double that to pay back Trevor as well.'

'Gees, they were great white boots though, Dave.'

And the Lee Hazlewood number, "These Boots Are Made For Walking" played around and around in my head.

38

SURROUNDED BY PURPLE

Mum lost her job at the Camberwell dress shop due to some interpersonal problems. Neither Dad nor I could understand why it had happened. It is likely that she said something inappropriate. Unfortunately, too few people are forgiving. From that point, old habits returned and a new cycle of dropping into the abyss commenced. As Mum deteriorated, Dad and I took up the slack.

The deterioration started with withdrawal and self-imposed isolation. For Mum, it was about survival, but that survival didn't include others. It was a downward spiral of self-absorption, a quest for the Holy Grail, an inward search of the one piece of the great mystery that would change her life. She must have responded to a Rosicrucian advertisement because her life became devoted to the 'I AM Society.' The Rosicrucians' theology is built on esoteric truths of the past concealed from the average man that provides insight into nature, the physical universe, and the spiritual realm. Exclusivity is ensured from the start; this extraordinary breakthrough is not to be grasped by anyone. Not the average man, no, only a few erudite people could possibly grasp the beliefs of this sect.

We were surrounded by purple. Everything was purple. Purple books with chapter headings and important sections in bold, upper case purple print were throughout the house. The mass of purple was nauseatingly disconcerting, and in the simple act of opening one of these books I would have a vertigo-like experience of my third eye being drawn out of my forehead. I wished I could summon a *one eyed, one horned, purple people eater* right out of the sky as sung in the lyrics of a popular rock tune of the day.

When she saw me reading one she snatched it away from me and spat out, 'You couldn't possibly understand this. You're only a child.' After that she didn't leave the books lying around; they were locked in a special drawer amongst her numerous exercise books. Each exercise book had page after page of her hand writing. Long passages had been copied verbatim from the purple books. This search for self, the 'I AM', obsessed her.

My bedroom was separated from my parents by a reasonably long corridor, but it was not long enough to avoid hearing their debates. Well... they were not really debates, more like a one-sided discussion once Mum entered her irrational space. It is possible that rational discussion occurred, but I mainly heard the irrational as the conversations became more absurd and louder.

'You haven't been called, Milton. You couldn't possibly understand this.'

She would stay up all night reading the purple, and she'd sleep all day. One night in winter I heard from their bedroom, 'Milton, can you turn down the electric blanket. I am too hot.' Dad had the dual control for the blanket his side of the bed. Only half awake he dutifully adjusted the heat control. Ten minutes passed and Mum threw off another blanket and then said, 'Milton, I am roasting, turn me down another notch.'

'There you go, Hazel.'

I dropped off into semi-sleep only to hear Mum again, 'Turn the thing off will you. I can't take any more and I've taken all the blankets off.'

We had become suspicious of her in so many ways and could have put the incident down to her instability, but this incident was not Mum's fault. The heat control box had been turned through one-hundred and eighty degrees, and Dad thought he was decreasing the heat when in fact he was increasing it. The discovery was made the next morning and Dad was telling me the story as he drove me to school. Wow, I thought, *The old man was trying to fry my mother.* Maybe he was trying to disrobe her to have some sex. It could be a good story to share with Dave and Trevor, but I was too reserved to speak about such things. There is no way that the Harrison family could speak with such candour and openness. We lived in a cloak of secrecy and acted as though everything was fine, all normal, nothing wrong here.

If you block out others, the only one left is God. And the harmonium played '*What A Friend We Have In Jesus.*' I mean, what a self-centred concept, the I AM Society, the emphasis on the 'I.' I exist. I am. What about the rest of us? Can you take some time out and think about that?

At the back of the house was a closed-in porch which contained a toilet. My bedroom was alongside the porch. I heard her fall in the toilet with a horrible sigh as air involuntarily escaped her lungs. Her medication imbalance and oscillations often left her constipated, and she had passed out after a protracted attempt at a bowel movement. I fetched Dad and we extracted her from the toilet. I understood the fragility of life. I had anger so big that I needed Robbie Flood back in my life. In the absence of Robbie, I developed an aggressive, antagonistic, contrarian streak. I struggled with the dichotomy of being an individual and the drive to be accepted by others.

Mum was a victim, a victim of circumstance. Life happened to her, passed her by, and became one to be suffered, endured. She was isolated, carved out, and separate. She had no counsellors, no confidant, no one with whom she could share emotions. She was stranded, unloved, and beached on the sands of her own making. It turns out there is Hell on earth.

The sadness still overwhelms me. It seeps into every room, occupies every object, but I cling to whatever remnants I have of hers even now. I stare in wonder at the three paintings I have of hers, all completed in her youth. The shed with the waterwheel turning in the stream amidst mossy rocks and a back lit sky could have been a cover for George Eliot's '*The Mill on the Floss.*' There is the one of tangled salmon gums alongside a shoreline in some exotic Asian locale with a prince's castle in the background. It has a serene mystical appeal that could have adorned the cover of M.M. Kaye's '*The Far Pavilions.*' But my favourite remnant of hers is the mother polar bear protectively astride her baby cub on an ice raft appropriately titled '*Adrift.*' To paint this, she must have had strong maternal instincts at the time.

She had so much talent, so much promise and creativity. I weep for the loss of a life of greatness that she may have led if not afflicted with her chemical imbalance and the ignorance of the times to identify her affliction and bring her back into normality. I have elaborately framed a print of Gari Melcher's 1904 painting of a mother and child. It hangs in our bedroom. I acquired the print as a freebie inducement from an encyclopaedia salesman. Gari Melcher, an American son of a German sculptor, was of the Dusseldorf School of painting. The painting is exquisite in its detail and reveals so much in the eyes of the mother. Hope, pride, nurture, acceptance in the face of disappointment, not knowing, and fear are all expressed here in the eyes. The child is a picture of complete innocence. The final message is, 'This child is mine and woebegone anyone that harms my child.'

Hazel must have passed through, must have experienced the Melcher mother's passions. Surely, she started out like that, but what went wrong? She was broken, snapped in two, and could not reassemble. She could have painted on and said so much, but her life stopped. Reluctantly, she gave birth to two sons and abandoned them and her husband causing misery to all and sundry. She was the problem and played but a small part in the solution through reluctant service. This seems harsh as I write it, and I wish to retract it, but I leave it as I search and stumble towards a semi-truth that I can come to understand. I never understood, and Dad never understood, the world she retreated into.

Was I ever nourished at her breast? I will never know. Brian cannot recall. Dad is dead. Aunt Joy died three months and three days short of a hundred. It was not the sort of question I could ask my ASIO trained Aunt. Institutional secrecy layered upon generational secrecy. To talk of such things is outlandish, the horror of horrors. There is little doubt in my mind that Mum would have suffered postnatal depression so I may have been taken from her care early on for reasons of safety, but I will never know.

****

Dad carried the load for the family. At the age of seventy-four he eventually drowned in his congestive bronchial grief. His heart could not clear the lifetime of cumulative tears that had collected in his lungs. It was all very sudden, a massive heart attack in the small hours of the night. Mum kept looking for the purple answers in the little Rosicrucian books, searching for the cryptic pathway to salvation, to Nirvana, to deliverance. Deliverance from what to where? Deliverance from reality into a bottomless spiritual haven where all would be well, a human fantasy constructed under the auspices of the all-powerful God?

Hazel's world had shrunk, becoming smaller and smaller. I believe in expansion, growth, development. I detest stagnation. Keep mobile, dance, and be free. Develop, develop, expand, and continue to grow. Believe in that and you can survive. Resources abound and are a function of man's creativity - explore and go forth to find them. I became a geologist.

Mum's illness arose when she became locked in her own mind, a shrinking mind with fewer opportunities. She needed to embrace the universal mind. The universal mind, God, is the body of us all as a collective, and if that premise is accepted then there is not one universal truth. The importance of friends to avoid the pit of eternal flame, the burning abyss is so obvious if you have looked into the abyss. Man cannot get there alone nor survive alone. Solitary confinement is a cruelty beyond measure. Man is a group animal. Find your group and plug in. Maybe even the insanity of bouncing up and down at a rock concert helps an individual to survive.

****

Religion offers man a reason to live and a reason to die. We seek to understand life and are not here simply to eat and reproduce. There is life beyond mere worldly sustenance, leisure, and pleasure. Without a cause, what is the point of mere existence? Our spirituality is what makes us rise above an ordinary animalistic life. Religion defines in cryptic language the importance of love, compassion, and the consideration of 'other' to fight against selfishness and destructive powers associated with the delusions of wealth.

I have personally experienced the double-edged sword that is religion. For Mum, it drove her into isolation. The solitary meditator may be driven to insanity. Religion only serves if it drives towards and embraces the 'other', a broad community. If the so formed community is driven by 'Onward Christian Soldiers' we generate another problem. That problem is only overcome through tolerance and respect for all.

****

At the height of unwellness is a lack of feeling. The sufferer is insensitive, unaware of people, events, places, and history. Extremes of behaviour, whether of dullness or fury, prevent feeling and the sufferer takes their own shortcomings out on whomever they are closest to. I now ask myself, why didn't I confront Mum? Why did I treat her like a porcelain doll that could shatter at any moment? No. I accepted her permanent dullness and never challenged her. In the end, I felt I had no relationship with her. There were too many taboo topics mixed up between mental illness and ASIO family secrecy. The tragedy is haunting, haunts me yet, and it's bloody painful.

39

ALMOST ALL OVER RED ROVER

It was Easter. Trevor and I had just started our university studies while Dave was making money in retail. His ambition was to one day own a shop. By now he had his first car, an FJ Holden. They had a reputation of being a bit scatty, light in the rear, and easy to fishtail out of control. We planned a hunting trip to Orbost in East Gippsland but were of an age that planning details were sparse. Alfred Siedlecki, a Polish friend from our high school, was to have been with us but was a late withdrawal due to coming down with the flu. In hindsight, it turns out that he was lucky to catch the virus.

We set off early and made Leongatha by eight o'clock and up until Leongatha our wit was low, but after having bought some cola and chips we came alive.

'I want to do some real driving now,' Dave announced.

We left the main highway and took a dirt road that headed towards Foster. The road was on the right side of a ridge as we drove east, and beneath us the grassy slope fell away over three hundred feet into a deep valley. Friesian dairy cattle grazed on the tree denuded slopes. I was in the front passenger seat alongside Dave, and Trevor was in the back seat. The warmth of the sunrise, the cola, and the dramatic scenery had transformed our earlier lethargy. Trevor belched, and Dave and I ribbed him about being a slob.

It happened quickly. Dave lost control of the car, and the FJ started fishtailing down the road. One moment I was looking at a cliff face, the next I was looking out into blue sky. Dave was frantically wrenching the steering wheel from side to side. Cliff face, sky, cliff face, sky, cliff face, sky, and then BANG! The left-hand fender clipped the cliff face, and the car was shunted towards the other side of the road. The right back wheel was over the edge and the car sat suspended, motionless, hanging in space. At that very moment, if I had had the gumption, I could have simply opened the door and stepped out of the car.

However, you don't leave your mates, do you? The car commenced to roll.

Mr Cool, Dave, said one word, 'Relax.' I don't know what else we could have done. For the first roll, it was easy to brace with arms and legs spread out. The second roll was quicker and more violent as the car gathered speed. The noise was immense and intruded above everything else.

I thought, This is it. My life is over, surely, I will not survive.

I awoke with a thud as I landed on my back. The damp of lush wet grass penetrated my shirt. My feet were facing down the hill and I passively watched the car rolling over its axis, hitting the ground and then bouncing in the air. It was Dam Buster like behaviour bouncing on the steep slope. The hollow thump of metal on earth, as if a boxer was hit in the solar plexus, was accompanied by the shrill tinkle of shattering glass.

'Bang, tinkle tinkle, bang, tinkle tinkle, impact, crunch, bounce, bounce,' the car leaped towards the valley floor.

The car stopped with a final rock from side to side, three hundred feet below after it had nowhere else to go. I looked at the wispy clouds passing, like angels, across the blue sky. I felt my arms and legs, testing to make certain they moved. They did. I passed my hand across my face, around my head, and through my hair. No blood. I sensed movement on the slope above me. It was Dave.

'You okay, Dave?'

'Yeah, I think so. How about you?'

'Yeah.'

I stood up, and there was Dave about fifteen feet above me. He stood holding his hand, and he had his shoulders drawn around towards his chest. Apart from that he looked alright.

'Trevor's still in the car,' he said.

I could now see Trevor's blonde-haired head some seventy-five feet way below, stark against the lush green.

'Trevor, are you alright?' I yelled.

There was no movement and he didn't answer. I yelled again, 'Trevor! Are you alright?'

There was a slight movement and we heard a quiet reply, 'Yes.' It was little above a whisper. It was now silent, and our ears were attuned to the acute awareness of even the rustle of leaves and the wonder of life after near death. Dave and I, without another word, lay back on the ground thankful that Trevor had survived.

'We can't lie like this all day. Let's go and see Trevor,' Dave said. As he reached me he added, 'One car down the piss.'

'We're bloody lucky to be alive,' I muttered.

'I'm sorry. If it was my fault, I'm sorry. Do you think it was my fault?'

'It just happened,' was all I could think of to say with no solace in my voice.

We reached Trevor who was now sitting up with one leg extended and holding his ankle.

'How are you, mate?'

'Bloody sore all over, and my bloody ankle is swelling up.'

'Give us a look,' I said. I could feel myself shaking as he slowly took off his shoe and a sock. It was badly swollen.

'Hell, it doesn't look too bloody good. It could be broken,' I said.

'I think it'll be alright,' he responded.

'The thing is we are alright. You stay here, and we'll go and have a look at the car,' Dave said, taking control of the situation.

It wasn't a pretty sight. The roof had been flattened to be level with the bonnet. The driver's side front wheel was at right angles to the body, hanging like a thread. The boot lid was open, bent along a diagonal axis, and the boot itself was bare of all contents apart from a four-gallon drum of petrol. The two doors on the driver's side were open and distorted but remarkably still attached to the car. There was no remnant of any window glass and the right-hand indicator light was blinking at us, infuriatingly making a click-click noise.

'There you go. I indicated I was doing a right-hand turn,' Dave quipped.

I managed a perfunctory laugh.

Dave walked over to the distorted drum of petrol, lifted it away from the car and screwed the lid off. Petrol blew out of the can ten foot into the air due to the contained pressure. He screwed the cap back on and rewrapped his hanky around his hand. All his knuckles were weeping like a boxer's after a fight.

Dave said the obvious, 'The car's a write off. Let's get out of here.'

We walked up to Trevor, who had his shoe back on, and found he could walk. We stumbled back up the slope to the road. It was like a bomb scene. We discovered Dave's rifle, the barrel bent in a semi-circle. Chops and sausages were spread everywhere soon to be food for dingoes and crows. Our three personal packs that were in the boot were ejected as one as though tied with rope and sat neatly together and upright. We hoisted them onto our backs. For some inane reason, we scanned the hillside for our cigars.

'There they are,' Dave said.

We heard a car on the road way up above us, then we saw it. I prayed it would stop. It did, and two heads appeared over the road verge.

'Vatt has happened?' one man asked. 'You roll over?'

'Anyvun hurt?' the other asked.

'Na, all good,' Dave replied.

'Gee, you boys vas very lucky. Come, I give you a hand.'

The two men descended from the road and gave us a hand with our packs, helping us get through the wire boundary fence to the paddock.

'Come boys, I'll take you back to the farm.'

He was driving an old tray back utility truck. We threw our packs onto the tray back and tentatively climbed aboard. Our hesitancy was due in part to the Alsatian dog sitting in the tray.

'He is very friendly. He vill keep you company.'

I had a vice like grip on the board behind the driver's cabin, and alternated between looking over the edge back into the valley and the slobbering face of the Alsatian whose teeth were far too visible. Also, his breath turned my stomach. In between times I glanced at Dave and Trevor, their faces white and expressionless.

The truck turned off onto a lesser track and we reached a farmhouse. A rather buxom but attractive woman opened the kitchen door.

'Come in, come in. You vill have a cup of coffee.' The woman stated it as fact rather than a question.

After we had told our story, I noticed she added some brandy to our coffees and then she said, 'You vill have some sugar in your coffee if you like it or not. It is good.' She placed three heaped teaspoons in each mug.

They were very concerned about Trevor. They thought he was showing signs of shock, so he was banished to a bedroom to rest. He looked fine to me. With his blonde hair and fair complexion, he always looked pale. Trevor was none too pleased and protested.

'I can't help it if I haven't got a ruddy complexion like you country folk,' he muttered.

'No, this one has a touch of shock,' said the other man who picked us up. 'I've seen quite a few shock cases in my time during the war.'

'Yes, I think you are right,' the lady said. Trevor lost the battle and he was led to lie down in a bedroom.

The brandy was very effective at settling Dave and I down. It was decided that we should drive back to the scene of the accident to see what could be done. When we arrived, there were two other young men climbing back up the hillside. They had been down to the wreckage. These boys had been out working the cows on the other side of the valley and had seen the accident.

'Gawd, you all survived! Bloody miracle,' one of the young men said.

'Where's their blonde-haired mate, the one that went around about eight times?'

'He's back at the farm lying down. Got a bit of shock,' responded the farmer.

'Do tell. He should be ringing the bell at church after this.' He continued, 'We saw the whole thing. The car was just hanging there and then it started to roll. It was a perfect roll on the long axis of the car. It hit the ground just before the fence and then it cleared the fence. Every time it hit the ground the doors sprang open and a body dropped out and the car would just go over the top. The driver came out first, then the next guy came out, and the poor bugger in the back seat, the blonde one, had to rattle around all that extra time in the car. You see they all came out of the front driver's door. It's a bloody miracle, I tell ya. You can count each roll because there is a dent of ripped up grass where the car bounced.'

And with that, he came over all emotional and embraced us.

'You guys were so lucky there are no trees in that paddock,' the farmer said.

'Not only that. You would have been goners if you were wearing seat belts. You would have ridden the car to the bottom,' said the other emotive young man.

The other man spoke for the first time, 'The car's a write off. We'll give you twenty pounds for it. We can use the wheels for a trailer and if the engine's any good we might be able to use it on the farm or drop it in a fishing boat.'

Dave, although looking miserable, responded, 'Make it twenty-five and it's yours.'

'Deal.' They shook on it.

If Dave could negotiate from this state of weakness, I knew he'd succeed in business.

✳✳✳✳✳✳✳✳✳

Back at the farmhouse, we had a grand lunch of pickled pork, potatoes, sauerkraut, and more brandy laden coffee. We were later driven into Leongatha to catch the train back to Melbourne. We didn't say much on the return other than to say repeatedly, 'Gees, we're lucky.'

'Yeah, we were. Better buy a raffle ticket when we get back.'

'Not wrong there. Gees, we were lucky.'

We parted at Spencer Street station and made our way home to surprise our parents and tell the story all over again.

'Gees, you were lucky, son. You're meant for greatness. I reckon you could be prime minister one day,' my father proclaimed, more out of habit than conviction.

40

BECOMING A GEOLOGIST

I became a geologist by accident. Back in the sixties, biochemistry was attracting many a young budding scientist. Given that chemistry was one of my strengths I was attracted to it, however, I had the fortune to be interviewed by the Dean of Science, himself a geologist, and he suggested I at least enrol in Geology I. I loved the subject.

What a contrast from my early ambitions of becoming a mathematician. Geology is an eclectic science which borrows from all the sciences to build its body of knowledge. There are lots of theories, few absolutes, and even fewer proofs. It is based on observation and description including both deductive and inductive reasoning, all under great uncertainty. All can be questioned, so it is forever alive. Geology demands engagement with both nature and academia, requiring an ability to present, defend, and debate a case.

Thankfully, I had always been an avid reader. I still am, as like most things if it becomes a habit in your developmental years then it stays with you for life. Just as well because countless hours had to be spent in the library reading the multitude of subject material embraced within the science of geology. I had yet to discover the philosophic insight of "what you see in the macrocosm is reflected in the microcosm." This concept was to come to me much later in life. Study is required at the microscopic level to the megascopic levels of mountain formation and continental drift, to name but two. The following subjects arranged from the micro to the macro were studied - crystallography, petrology and petrography, mineralogy, geochemistry, palaeontology, sedimentology, stratigraphy, geomorphology, geophysics, structure and tectonics, and economic geology.

This is such a broad range of material, what do you study? I was driven mainly by curiosity as the material was all new and interesting to me. The learning was anything but linear. There was no guarantee that you were studying the right material, lots of dead ends were reached, and searches undertaken. You were on your own, left to your own devices. This was not prescribed learning; there were no guarantees. It was an exploration, much like the career to come. This was all done by taking lots of notes. I cannot remember even submitting that many assignments. Interspersed between lectures and reading, whatever you could get your hands on in the library were three-hour practicals in rock, mineral, fossil, and petrographic microscope work. Of course, it was essential to be competent and pass the practicals.

The other necessary practical work was field excursions to understand the mega-form in which rocks present themselves. Ultimately, field mapping assignments were done as exercises. This was to prepare us for the ultimate requirement of "field work" once we graduated into the work force.

Progress from one year to the next was dependent upon passing the annual three-hour examination papers.

Student attrition was high with approximately sixty or more undertaking Geology I, but by year three, there were only twenty brave souls studying Geology III. Attrition from the industry afterwards is even more rapid. Of our 1967 graduation class, only four stayed in the profession for more than ten years. Field work demands, economic recessions, matrimonial demands, or lifestyle restrictions all took their toll. Being a small group and participating in field excursions together made for some great friendships and camaraderie.

Because of my school sporting achievements, I thought I would be a walk-in start up with the Uni Blues Aussie rules side, but despite regularly training I was overlooked. This was a body blow for the ego. I defended my ego through the justification that the Uni Blues was run by an in-group of ex-private school players and I was from the state high school system. In my maturity, I now understand that the universe doesn't make mistakes. I simply took up other pursuits and joined Judo and the University Mountaineering Club. The latter of course was a good fit for my future career as a geologist as I participated in rock-climbing, speleology, camping out, and bush-walking. With respect to the former, I didn't advance beyond a "yellow" belt – didn't like the "strangle-holds!"

The most memorable university lecturer we had was Professor O P Singleton, otherwise known as OPS. The man was an inspiration. His soft-rock subjects of palaeontology, sedimentology, and stratigraphy were given with great passion and humour. His lectures on European stratigraphy contained exquisite detail on soil types overlying key rock-types that impacted the quality of French wines. I couldn't bring myself to throw away my stratigraphy uni notes until I decided to retire from geology after forty-six years in the profession. At last, I was beginning to see some utility in studying geology. As brilliant as he was, he was one of the last leading world-renowned geologists to not accept continental drift. He would dig up palaeontologic details to refute the theory. Of course, this theory has now been subsumed by plate tectonics.

OPS had an amazing and impractical academic's office. Each wall was lined with book cases. He had one large dining table placed in the centre of the room with lots of books just stacked in individual piles on it. This battleground represented both his filing and reference system. There was no spare surface anywhere that I could see upon which he could write.

This era was basically pre-computers. During my university years, there was one main frame computer in the chemistry building which took up one large, laboratory-size room. I did not even own a calculator nor, unlike the engineering students of the day, a slide rule. My pride and joy was a book of five-figure logarithms. There were some determined souls playing with computers, designing programmes using a system of "punchcards" which recorded the on-off switches for the data input. I was not one of the enthusiasts. My growth in computing as a user was a lengthy process throughout my career. A lot of front-end effort was required before there was an adequate return for the invested time. The returns were minimal back then, and involvement with it was a drag on doing the job or advancing the project at hand.

In this pre-computer era, all notes remained handwritten. Assignments could be submitted hand written, filing systems were card systems, calculations were manual assisted by logarithmic look-up tables, and the mobile phone had not yet been invented. Compare this with today. Spread-sheeting allows each of us to do complex mathematical manipulations and design illustrative graphs. Word processing allows for the cutting and pasting of activities with automatic spell-check. "Google Search" on the Internet has given each of us wonderful research access to material and publications. All the above, together with other sophisticated software, allow us to develop relational databases, detailed project plans, and open up all sorts of possibilities of individuals relating to each other.

Without these tools back in the mid-1960s we had to know and learn how to seek out information in a more personal way. Interpersonal, face to face question and answer skills had to be developed. Listening skills had to be sharp as you would only get one chance at gathering data - no computer backup. No spell-check, so learn how to spell properly through understanding Latin roots to words, and tackling of complex mathematical problems from first principals and developed theories. No trusting the spreadsheet back then, and always verify the final answer, now we call it output, through crosschecking. Express yourself carefully with sufficient prior thought when writing by hand as correction is difficult, time consuming, and quite ugly when presenting results with too many crossed out sections in a final product. No PowerPoint presentations back then, so learn to verbalise and describe fully with much arm-waving and fewer illustrations.

Poverty is a relative term. Compared to today's student I was poor. No doubt I was better off than many of the other students, but I certainly didn't have much spare money. I was still living in my parent's home and classified as a dependent. Yes, I had won a Commonwealth Scholarship to attend university, however, benefits were means-tested so I did not receive any weekly allowance. The scholarship just entitled me to an annual book allowance and fee free education. I am forever grateful to my parents. I did not have to pay any board, so I had the safety of a roof over my head, healthy food, and support. The job at Des Casey's provided petty cash.

What income I did have I spent mainly on books, as this was a period of rapid expansion of my knowledge and understanding of all sorts of things. I had a catholic, voracious appetite and read widely. I had left school with a recommended reading list of good literature supplied by the English teacher and I worked my way through the list. I even contemplated becoming a writer. I would keep a record of interesting quotes from books and I always had a notebook in my top pocket.

Other expenses were on social activities and transport. I played cricket with the Camberwell Sub-District third eleven in the summer months. In fact, I captained the third eleven for two seasons. Cricket was a great joy and passion. About this time, or a little earlier, I bought my first trombone. Little was I to know that the trombone would ultimately become an important part of my life. Socially, I was a one-pot screamer simply because I had such little money. How could you afford the second pot? I dabbled with smoking. Filter-less Pall Malls and Camels were the favoured brands, and as I was going through my pretend mathematics professor, not of this world, writer, academic, image phase, I smoked pipes for a period. It was never very heavy as I was again limited through a lack of income. In hindsight, how lucky was I?

41

LUCKY RABBIT LUCKY DENNIS

It was another wet, drizzly Saturday morning in Melbourne and Dave, Trevor, Alfred, and I were heading off for the June Queen's Birthday long weekend to do some hunting. We departed from Elwood at six in the morning in Alf's Hillman Minx loaded with food, camping equipment, and guns.

I certainly hoped this trip would be less dramatic than the earlier Easter hunting trip. That trip had resulted in Dave's car being written off, but at least no lives had been lost.

I had befriended Alf in my last year at Elwood High School and had broken him into the long-established trio that was Dave, Trevor, and I. Alf wanted to be accepted into our group as a fair dinkum Aussie.

We were all a little sleepy on the drive because of the early hour of our departure, but the light banter soon started.

'Hey Seeds, how are you getting on with Michelle Frydenberg?' I asked.

Trevor added, 'Yeah, spreading any of those seeds of yours yet, Alf?'

'Ya, Ya, she very nice girl,' Alf responded as he drove with one hand on the wheel, looking behind to reply to Trevor and I. We had quickly sat in the back seat upon departure after our earlier Easter experience with Dave at the wheel.

'She's one hell of a hot bird, Alf. You lucky dog,' I teased.

'I no dog. I good Polak boy,' Alf responded.

'Sure Alf, you'll make a good enough Aussie one day,' I went on.

By now we were navigating through the back streets of North Melbourne before setting off towards Bacchus Marsh, situated some fifty kilometres west of Melbourne. Animatedly, Alf turned his head and tapped his amply large nose with one finger as he spoke, 'She very good Jewish girl, you know what I mean ………….'

'ALF, on your RIGHT!' yelled Trevor.

Too late, Alf planted both feet forward, the brakes locked, and as though in a slow motion replay the car slid straight into the other vehicle.

BANG! It's always the noise that gets to you in an accident. We all stepped out from the car, it was only the car that had been damaged. Alf was very sheepish with nowhere to hide: it was his fault. Trevor and I were shaking as it had only been two months prior that Dave had written off his car on the Easter hunting trip. Alf's car had its right headlight out of its mounting and hanging by an electrical lead, and the fender had been forced onto the front tyre. It was obvious that the car could not be driven away. I was having thoughts of maybe I would have to spend the rest of the weekend on that University assignment with the looming deadline.

'Tell you what, you guys stay with Alf and help him with the clean-up. I'll catch a taxi, get my car, and we can still go hunting,' said Dave, the man of steel, who took accidents in his stride due to his considerable experience. He was the wealthiest of the four of us as he was the only one not studying and in the workforce. He had already replaced his car from the Easter 'incident.'

'Great idea,' agreed the forever loyal Trevor and I without hesitation.

'Yes, okay,' Alf managed to get out. 'It just slid out there you know.'

We consoled Alf as he sadly watched his car being towed away.

Alf was a big bear of a man who could have just stepped out of a Siberian forest. Alfred Siedlecki was in fact a Polish Jew, his family having emigrated from Podlaise, a north-eastern province of Poland. We called him either Alf or 'Seeds.' Stripped to his shorts and athletic singlet he looked enormous, making any pubescent adolescent girl sigh and most young men mentally note not to mess with him. He was a shoe-in for the shot put, discus, and javelin at the school sports each year. No one could match Alf. Naturally given his origins, he was an outstanding chess player and could play a powerful and strategic game of tennis. He was also a brilliant mathematician and an emerging young scientist. I had kept in touch with him since we had graduated from Elwood High School.

'It was slow you know, it just slid out there,' Alf kept repeating.

'We know. Could happen to anyone, mate.' I did my best to console him.

Through the sheeting rain, steel man Dave eventually arrived in his latest FJ Holden replacement and all the gear was transferred.

'Take two boys, let's get into the rabbits,' Dave said as we took off again.

We had all become a little quiet. Dave was doing his best to lift our spirits. Alf was morose and just kept repeating, 'It was so slow, it just slid right out there.'

It was still raining when we hit Bacchus Marsh an hour later, and as we had lost so much time, there was nothing to do but have lunch.

'Lads, let's go and have a counter-lunch at the pub,' Dave suggested, 'Too much rain to do anything else anyway.' There was complete enthusiasm to that decision. Pie, chips, and several beers later, we were a much happier travelling party, especially since there was a break in the rain.

'We had better hoof it off to Lerderderg State Park and set up camp while we can,' Dave said. We arrived at the park within the hour, and selected our camp site to setup our tents.

'There is just enough time for a dusk shoot and scout, lads. The maps show there is a good flat area along the floodplain of the creek just over that little ridge. Grab your guns, and a shoulder bag to bring home the loot,' said Dave optimistically. He had the most experience with guns by far.

We set off chatting about how we would cook the rabbit stew until we hit the ridge where we were forced to reduce to single file, and then we walked in silence.

The silence was broken by an almighty 'BANG'.

'What the... Jesus... You dumb Polak! You could have blown off my leg.' I yelled. I looked down at a fist-size crater an inch away from my right foot.

'Bloody hell Seeds... You could've killed him,' Trevor chipped.

'See that thing there Alf, it's called a safety catch. You keep it on at all times, until you see a rabbit,' Dave instructed. 'Let's head back to camp. We've frightened any rabbits away now.'

'Sorry, sorry,' a chastened Alf managed to get out.

Back at camp we prepared our evening meal.

'Hey, Alf. What's in the bottle?' I asked.

'Ogorki Kiszone,' Ralph said, 'made by my Matka.'

I responded, 'Don't come the Polish sausage with me Alf.'

As he replied Alf pulled out some smoked Polish sausage, some sauerkraut, and a bottle of Vodka, 'You dumb Aussie. I show you how to eat.'

'This very good Vodka, Chopin Vodka, not cheap, top shelf,' Alf proudly explained. 'It made from potatoes grown in Podlaise. That's where I come from, ya! Seven pounds of potatoes go into every bottle.' He went on as he produced four small glasses and poured out the vodka, 'This is how you eat the Ogorki Kiszone.' At that he selected a dill pickle, took a large bite, and then tossed down a glass of vodka. 'There you go, now your turn.' We all followed suit.

The fire water hit our stomachs and brought tears to our eyes, temporarily stealing our voices.

'It good, ya. We go again,' said Alf, rolling his sleeves up.

'This real good, plenty of garlic too. Don't eat these alone if you're with Michelle, mate. Make sure she is eating them too,' said Trevor, forever helpful.

Alf became all reflective as he thought of Michelle, his damaged car, and maybe even nearly shooting me. The others could see he might drop into his morose talk of 'it just slid out there' again and Trevor jumped in, 'You'll make a good Aussie one day, Alf.'

'Ya, I marry Michelle and I make little Polaks.'

'No, you marry Michelle and make little Aussies,' Trevor said.

'Ya, little Aussie Polaks.'

'I reckon you'll be a rocket scientist one day, Alf,' Trevor continued.

'Ya, and I'll fire them towards Moscow.' Alf was coming alive again.

'Didn't Chopin write some music?' I chimed in as he rolled the vodka bottle in his hands.

'You dumb, ignorant antipod. Chopin was the world's greatest Romantic composer and he was Polish,' Alf said as he snapped off some more dill pickle and threw another vodka shot down.

'Gees, your bloody sophisticated, Alf. That's what you are... sofist ee cated.' Then after a small pause I added, 'Not much of a driver though, got a bit of a problem with a gun too.'

'You're a bloody dill, Dennis,' Trevor said, forever the peace maker. At least he was smart enough to know that Alf was capable of tearing every limb away from my torso.

'What else you got in these pickles? I'm feeling a bit light headed,' I said.

'You're pissed, Dennis. Listen lads, lets get to bed and I'll get you up early for a dawn shoot in the paddock on the floodplain,' Dave said.

He was the natural leader and we deferred to his recommendation.

True to his word, Dave woke us before dawn. Sleepily, we soon emerged from our tents. The camp site wasn't pretty, strewn as it was with all the empty bottles.

'Get your guns. Alf, keep that bloody safety catch on. Now listen up, this is how we do it once we hit the paddock. We form a straight line across the paddock and then we quietly and slowly advance. No one gets ahead of anyone else, look across the line, and always know where everyone else is. Got it?' Dave instructed.

'Got it,' three voices responded in unison.

Soberly and slowly we set off, last night's incident still fresh in our minds, with eyes scanning forward, searching for prey and sideways looking at each other. We were all keeping a close eye on Alf.

Only fifteen minutes of time had lapsed but it seemed like an eternity of intense concentration for us fledgling hunters, when Dave held up his hand to stop. He then raised it to his lips as he mouthed the word, 'Shh!' He was pointing forward, and sure enough there was a rabbit. Dave indicated that we should raise our guns and take aim. Dave, Trevor, and I managed to get a single shot off. Alf just kept firing shot after shot. He had a 'Random Hunter' semi-automatic version of the AKM rifle. Nobody had hit the rabbit, it dodged left, it dodged right, and here's the crazy thing, it was running towards us. Dave's 'safety meeting' hadn't prepared us for this contingency. Alf just kept continually firing and lowering his rifle as the rabbit came closer and closer and then broke our line and ran between Alf and me. This didn't stop Alf. He just span around as though he was throwing the discus in the school sports and kept firing. Alf was out of control. Dave, Trevor, and I hit the ground. We didn't get up until Alf stopped shooting.

'Whoa big boy! Did you get him?' Trevor asked.

'Na, Na. Idiota, Idiota,' responded Alf, slapping his head with beads of sweat pouring off his face as though he had indeed been competing in the discus.

'Listen, you bloody Polak. You could have told us you had a bloody Kalashnikov,' I said once I could find my voice.

'Might just get back to camp guys, you normally only ever get one chance at the kill, the rabbits are all in their burrows now,' said Dave.

'Every responsible mother of anything that can bloody breathe has locked up all their offspring,' I muttered.

Shaking and subdued, we returned to camp.

'I think we might have had enough hunting school for now guys, might be a good idea to pack up after breakfast and get home. What do you say?' Dave suggested.

'Yeah. Alf, you got anymore of Matka's dill pickles?' Trevor asked.

'Na, Na. I go home and see Michelle now,' Alf responded.

'How are you going to do that Alf? You haven't got a car,' I jibed as I reaffirmed I still had an ankle by stroking it with my right hand.

Without missing a beat, the forever bighearted Dave said, 'You can take mine. You've graduated, Alf. You're one of us now.'

I couldn't be that generous.

42

ANOTHER NEAR MISS

Dad bought me a car near the end of my first year at university, a 1952 Fiat 500. This was a generous act. Whether he thought it safer than me running around in Dave's new FJ Holden or he could see the amount of time I was spending on travel I could only guess. 1952 was the last year that Fiat placed the engine in the front of their '500' range. It was a petite two-door car, coloured green with two green leather bucket seats and a very small bench behind. In the Australian vernacular it had been dubbed "Mighty Mouse."

It was the occasion of another inspirational speech from Dad. 'As captain of the third eleven you need something to run around in. If you drink and drive you're a bloody mug and not long for this world. Watch your drinking. You'll never make prime minister if you keep up that heavy drinking. Booze has been the downfall of many a man. I want to see you sitting on the green leather, son. Make a difference to this world. Give it a go.'

'Thanks, Dad. I'll give it a go,' I replied but in my mind, I was already sitting on the green leather bucket seats.

Two of my very good friends, Sam Snell and Frank Marsh, whom we called 'Swamp', both had cars. Sam had a Hillman Minx and Frank had a Ford Prefect. As we all lived in the eastern suburbs and finished afternoon practicals together we would regularly have a race home down Johnston Street through Fitzroy and Collingwood. Johnston Street was a busy road shared by trams heading due east from the university. None of our cars were power machines so victory was achieved through making the right traffic decisions. Mighty Mouse had its share of victories, and some of those came at the expense of double-declutch breakdowns. Instead of a universal joint Mighty Mouse had a fabric disc at either end of the drive shaft, held together with counter directional bolts. A double-declutch gear change if not done well could put a shudder through the car and undue strain on the fabric disc resulting in a breakdown.

Back in the 1960s you were either a rocker, a jazzer, or a surfie. I belonged to the "Jazzer" cult. One of my favourite haunts was the jazz dance in a hall at 431 St Kilda Road. I became a member, complete with a medallion. Now with a flash car and a new front tooth (my grey tooth had been filed down to a stump and had a dazzling white cap glued onto the stump), maybe I had the chance of attracting a girl.

I was really into jazz, loved the music. My brother, by his late teens, had developed into a good jazz pianist and led his own band. I was naturally drawn to the excitement of Dixieland jazz and the setup of the three lead instruments, trumpet, clarinet, and trombone underpinned with the three rhythm instruments, piano, bass, and drums. In my mid to late teens and in an attempt to copy Brian, I tried to lure Dave and Trevor into getting some instruments with the ambition of forming a band. Dave was too much his own character to be tempted but Trevor chose the clarinet, an instrument to which I had been attracted. Reluctantly I said, 'Oh well, I'll get a trombone.'

It wasn't a particularly good trombone, but it was all I could afford at the time. It was a Boosey small bore peashooter made in 1930, before Boosey met Hawkes and started their famous 'Boosey and Hawkes' instruments. It came in a battered case with a small cup mouthpiece. Fortunately, the most important part of a trombone, the slide, was in good condition. However, it required old fashioned slide oil such that when you played it an apron was needed for protection, if you valued your clothes that is, because oil flew everywhere. It was such a small trombone that when I entered the music shop to purchase a 'How to Play' book, I selected the Treble Clef version tutorial. This was to be quite fortuitous later on in my fifties when I chose to join a brass band.

My band never came to be, it was simply a passion of mine not shared by my friends. Trevor gave up the clarinet within the first year so I bought it off him. I had tried to teach myself the trombone, but now armed with the clarinet I began clarinet lessons from a reed teacher, hauling myself off into the city every Saturday morning. After an intense year and still out of reach of playing 'The Golden Wedding', I moth-balled my musical ambitions in favour of my studies.

When at the 431 Club, I would mainly place myself up the front of the hall near the band to better hear the music and observe their mastery. Hanging behind the band was a fish net, and concealed behind that was the 'pash-pit', an area of scattered pillows and rugs embellished with the excuse of a coffee machine. Couples spent a lot of time there over their coffees and my concentration shifted away from the music and my eyes misted over and I thought, Maybe I should be trying just a bit harder here, and so I started the grand parade around the hall.

'Would you like to dance?' I asked.

'Sure,' she replied demurely.

I let myself go. I was sure I had never danced so well before.

'I'm Dennis.'

'Cheryl.' This girl was so talkative. She had one-word responses to everything.

The music stopped, and I asked, 'Can I run you home?'

'That would be nice,' she replied. 'I live at Windy Hill, near Essendon. Is that too far for you?'

'Not at all. Love to do it,' I replied. God, I am so new to this game. I had asked the questions in the wrong sequence. Should have established where she lived before inviting to take her home. Windy Hill is right over the other side of the large city of Melbourne. Still here we go.

We left the dance and walked to the car holding hands, exchanging the odd kiss.

We drove across town largely in silence, she wasn't the talkative type and I, apart from developing some sort of plan, had to concentrate on navigation. A pleasant, anticipatory, provocative silence descended on the car. Sharp images cut through my brain.

Cheryl broke the silence, 'My house is only two blocks away from here.'

'Well, it's not too late yet. You mind if we stop here for a moment?'

'Fine by me.'

Some serious kissing and petting took place which is not that easy in bucket seats, so I suggested that we move to the back seat, really the back bench. Rather ungracefully, we got out of the car, pushed the seats forward, and entered the back of the car. There was much excitement as I had never gone this far before, and while trying to disengage clothes from each other I extended my leg between the two bucket seats and tripped the hand brake. There was a reason this suburb was named Windy Hill, it was the hilly part of Essendon. The car started to gently roll backwards down the hill. I pulled myself up and de-fogged the condensation on the little rear window to look out. Forget getting to the steering wheel, it was behind one of the bucket seats, not much to do but ride it out. The car gathered some speed then turned into a driveway with a slight rise. One rear wheel dropped into a small garden ditch alongside the driveway, and the bumper bar hit a tree.

Sexual thoughts abandoned, us two love birds stepped out of the car.

'I think we've climaxed Cheryl. I'll get you home,' I laughed.

As I drove home, still a virgin, I was thinking, 'If the real thing is as exciting as this I might have to try harder.' Then later I reflected, Surfies have no taste in music, but they are bloody smart owning those panel vans.'

43

THE FANTA MUST HAVE BEEN OFF

I met my wife to be, Kathy, at the Bureau of Meteorology on Spring St, Melbourne. This was the Bureau's head office. She was the most attractive girl working in the NSW climate room, and I was a student working on university vacation. I hadn't had too many paydays in my life up until that point, only casual money from Des Casey's, but being employed in February 1966, experienced the conversion to decimal currency. I had a few beers at a farewell lunch with my workmates. I had wanted to invite her out for weeks but that required more courage than facing up to a pace man bowling fast bouncers at your head. Primed with Dutch courage, I invited her out in the afternoon of my very last day at the Bureau. The Moomba festival was going on in Melbourne at the time, and she said yes. What a thrill, we saw the play 'Brigadoon' playing that night in Fawkner Park.

I was very dry in the mouth after my swilling of too many beers at my farewell lunch, and all I could purchase at the musical was a Fanta. It did not mix well with my earlier libations. I could feel myself going green toward the end of the performance and my applause was becoming quite insipid. Kathy shared a flat with her cousin Ian, her close friend Jill, who also worked at the Bureau, and Jill's brother Bob in Punt Rd, South Yarra. Kathy's flat was only a short walk through parklands to get her home, but it was too distant for me to make in my weakened state without incident. Fortunately, Fawkner Park has some very big trees and we had not advanced very far when I said to Kathy,

'You will have to excuse me for a moment.' I disappeared behind a tree at great pace and heaved my heart out making some ungodly noises. Kathy was still there when I re-emerged from behind the tree patting my mouth with a hanky.

'Sorry about that,' I said, 'It was the Fanta, it must have been off.'

She took my hand and escorted me towards her flat, very gallant on my part. I was surprised how understanding, forgiving, and without reprimand she had been. Mind you, that level of forgiveness only happens to the single man and is rarely repeated once married. What a way to start a grand romance.

****

Maybe I was a bit eccentric back then. Mighty Mouse had been off the road for a protracted time - another double-declutch mishap. Kathy probably thought I was spinning her a yarn about having a car. Once Dad and I had finally made the car road worthy again I proudly announced to her,

'I'll pick you and Jill up from work on Friday.'

****

I saw them waiting together on Spring St, and I pulled into the curb right alongside them. Mighty Mouse was only a small car and they looked right over the top of it not for one moment thinking that this could be me. I blew the horn, a little squeaky thing, and it didn't twig with them that this was indeed me picking them up. I wound the window down and remonstrated,

'Hey, you two. Can I run you home?'

'Is that really you?' Kathy asked surprised.

With a deprecating laugh Jill asked, 'What sort of car is this?'

'It's a very powerful Fiat 500,' I responded. I pushed the passenger front seat forward and said, 'You'll have to get in the back there, Jill.'

'What? In there?' She loudly asked, her voice rising.

'Yes, it's okay. I've had girls in the back there before.' She raised her eyebrow and entered the car. The space was so small that there was no other way to get in. I knew just how awkward it could be because of my experience with Cheryl. Once she had folded into the car, Kathy could sit in the front seat.

'Do you think this can make it up Punt Rd hill?' Jill asked in a nervous voice.

I had typed up instructions for passengers for moments just like this. I leaned forward and recovered them from the glove box, handed it to Jill. It read;

Conditions of Travel in Mighty Mouse TW 288

A) *Physical condition of passenger*

Male: max height 5'11," max weight 11 stone
Female: max height 5'9," max weight 8 and half stone

B) *Mental condition of passenger*

This faculty is of the utmost importance to the performance of the car. Passenger must be relaxed and under no circumstances, no matter how demanding the provocation or how severe the strain, show any sign of anxiety. Self-conscious passengers are advised to seek alternative transport as this car suffers from a great deal of public scrutiny.

C) *Miscellaneous clauses*

i) *Any accidents are automatically deemed the fault of passengers as the driver's ability cannot be questioned.*

ii) *Passengers are requested to limit personal luggage to the bare essentials. Due regard and kind consideration will be given to passenger's dress due to extraordinary weather conditions. This clause is especially coined for female passengers as they suffer from the 'excess luggage allergy' much more than males. As to weather conditions for female passengers and their dress;*

a) *Summer attire – no objections will be levelled by the driver if bikinis are worn; in fact, this sort of thing is encouraged.*

b) *Winter attire – either an umbrella or coat but not both will be allowed entry into the vehicle. Passengers are advised to wear coats as if any heavy rain may fall the car's resistance to rain fails correspondingly (i.e.: the roof leaks), and as umbrellas tend to pierce the fabric roof of the car when opened inside the car (this is hard to avoid) the coat is the better choice of the two.*

To Be Evaporated
Dennis Harrison

'There's no mention of this car being capable of carrying three people,' Jill pointedly commented, still doubting that the car could climb Punt Rd hill. Mind you she wasn't in a position of strength now that she was trapped in the back of the car.

'I'll have you know that this is a convertible. The roof can fold back,' I said.

'Here we go girls. A ride of a lifetime.'

I gunned the car at the bottom of the Punt Rd hill, and with ever decreasing speed we assailed to the top. In my peripheral vision I could see Jill fearfully looking out the little rear window down the hill with considerable doubt of her survival.

Arriving at their flat, I parked the car and we all got out. Jill crossed herself.

'What are you doing that for? You're not even a Catholic?' said Kathy.

'I am all stiff from being in the back. Thanks for the lift Dennis but I think I'll catch the tram next time.'

'Could be right there, Jill. I think this is meant to be just a car for two.'

'Two love birds, hey,' she gibed.

'I think we all need a stiff drink,' Kathy offered, 'How about a marsala?' That was Kathy's idea of a stiff drink back then. Her other drink was a Pimm's but in all truth, she was not much of a drinker.

****

Kathy and I had arrived back at her flat at the same time as Ian and his girlfriend Julie. We were enjoying each other's company when we all felt like a hamburger, despite the late hour. Ian took charge.

'Now what would you like Julie?' Ian asked.

'You know I don't want any beetroot. It gets all over you, and definitely no garlic. Everything else is fine.'

'Right. And you, Kathy?'

'At this late hour I think I'll skip the egg and no onions.'

'Okay. And Dennis?'

'I'll come down with you and decide when I get there.'

'Fine. We won't be long girls,' Ian said.

The take away shop was only a hundred yards down the road.

We entered the shop surprised to see that it was packed with about ten customers. There was only one operator behind the counter, frantically working away.

'I had the army through here about an hour ago, bloody mayhem,' he said as he wiped his hands on his once white but now artistically multi-coloured besmirched apron.

'I can see,' Ian said. 'Looks like you've come from a MASH unit in Vietnam.'

'What?'

'Never mind.'

'What would you like?' he asked as he passed one hand though his Brylcreemed greasy hair that had deposits of sauce embedded within it.

'We want four burgers in all. One with the lot but no beetroot and no garlic. Put tomato sauce on that one. The second one, one with the lot but no egg and no onion, and put tomato sauce on that. I'll have one with no egg, no bacon, and barbeque sauce. What do you want, Dennis?'

'Make the fourth one with the lot and barbeque sauce, thanks.'

He wiped his hands across his apron, which made them even stickier, and elaborately took a pen from behind his ear, quickly scribbling the order down.

'There's a few people ahead of you so it'll be a little while. Had the bloody Army through here before, only an hour ago.'

'Fine, we're good to wait.' Ian responded and as an aside to me said, 'The army is used to eating in a mess.'

'What was that?'

'Nothing, nothing. I just said do your best.'

There was a great flurry of activity on his hot plate as he flipped patties, cracked eggs, and grilled onions. In between, he cut buns, spread butter, added lettuce, the occasional beetroot, and pineapple rings. He particularly enjoyed squirting the sauce from an elevated height in a flourish. He would then wrap up his creation in some grease proof paper.

Once a burger had reached the fully wrapped state he would assertively announce what it was, 'Plain burger with bacon and cheese and barbeque sauce.'

Many announcements were met with silence. Customers were getting restless and transferring their weight from one foot to the other. At this late hour, many of the customers were also a little worse for wear having arrived from parties of one sort or the other.

'No mate, I ordered a plain burger with bacon, no cheese, tomato sauce, and an egg.'

'Bugger it. I had the army through here an hour ago. They wait for no man you know. Well, there goes another one.' And with that he would pick the burger up and slam it with great force into a dust bin under the counter. 'We'll start again.'

Ian and I exchanged amused glances. We didn't wish to say too much in the shop because it could inflame the situation. Customers were agitated, and the shop keeper was unravelling before our eyes. He was run off his feet, his brain no longer thinking systematically. He may have been one step away from a mental breakdown. He would pause, wipe his hands on his apron, and with a sigh inquire, 'Now, what was your order?'

This played out before us repeatedly, 'Now what was your order?' He would have been better off just giving free burgers away instead of throwing them in the bin, but he insisted on getting the order exactly right. There was no profit in operating like this. It must have been over an hour and a half before we left the shop with our four burgers. I had been breathing the fumes of burning beef, eggs, and onions for so long that I was no longer hungry, but the entertainment had been much better than the show Kathy and I had seen earlier in the night. By the time it came to our burgers, whatever he had called out we claimed as ours.

We returned to the flat in hysterics. 'Now what was your order?' Ian mocked.

'What took you so long?' Julie innocently asked. And then we attempted to explain to the girls what had happened. Given the length of time we were away, the girls had one extra Pimm's too many and we were all rolling in laughter.

'Do you know I ordered one with no beetroot, no garlic, and tomato sauce. You got it all wrong. I've got one with beetroot and barbeque sauce,' Julie said.

This started us off again. 'Just be grateful, one, that you have a burger and two, that it was close to your order,' Ian responded.

The memory of this experience has travelled with the four of us undiminished throughout the years, and we cannot meet with each other without its ready recall.

44

OH NO A PURPLE SPORTS COAT

Kathy was a Victorian country girl, born in Maryborough. She enjoyed a carefree country upbringing that included horse riding, tennis, and dancing. As a result, she had a generosity of spirit and a genuine interest and care for people.

She obtained her Leaving Certificate from the Brigidine Convent and initially worked at the Maryborough Knitting Mills and, when eighteen, went to Melbourne to work at the Bureau of Meteorology. She boarded first at St Anne's Hostel in the city and later shared a flat with her workmate and good friend, Jill, and Cousin Ian. Her father was a leading trainer and driver of pacers and trotters. He had some wonderful horses, one of which went on to win an Interdominion. If he had a winner on the night at the Melbourne Showgrounds, and he had a winner most meets, the Committee would invite him and his family and friends to the Committee Room for drinks. Now as an impoverished student, I had trained myself to be a one pot screamer basically because I could not afford the second glass, so this was just magic.

They may have been country people, but they and their friends were shrewd. One evening, I had backed a quinella and won fifty dollars. For a university student, that's a large amount of money. I was approached by one of their 'friends' in the Committee room with the opportunity to buy a sports coat that they just happened to have with them. 'For you, seeing your friends with Kathy, you can have it for fifty dollars.' The night had advanced somewhat. I was capitalising on the free drinks and in the dimly lit, smoke filled room the coat looked like a good buy to me. In the sobering light of the next morning, however, I discovered that I had bought a purple coloured sports coat that was short in the sleeves and small across the shoulders such that it popped my arms out like a chimpanzee. I'd been done over. It was a great disappointment, and besides our house was already suffering from an overdose of purple.

She had a flat and I had a car, great ingredients to assist the blossoming romance. Our attachment to each other was put to an early test. Kathy had been working at the Bureau for three years and had accumulated a tidy sum of money, enough to contemplate a trip overseas on a liner, the *Oriana*. This came as a huge surprise to me and I was none too pleased. I didn't want to see this girl that I had fallen in love with disappear overseas only to maybe meet some moneyed Pom or suave Italian. The *Oriana* was docked in the Port of Melbourne, and Kathy had four complimentary passes to board the ship. She had invited Ian, Julie, and I to accompany her. We drove independently to the port as Ian and Julie had plans to drive to Geelong afterwards. As they were about to leave I felt for the keys to Mighty Mouse in my pocket and couldn't find them.

'I must have left them in the car.' I broke out into a sweat.

'I'll go down with you and help you search for them,' Ian offered. The car was not locked, and we searched all over it, sliding the two bucket seats forward and back, looking under the mats, behind the sun visor. We even emptied out the glove box. I put the fabric roof back as well, to throw more light into the car. I was getting in quite a state.

Ian finally asked, 'Have you checked all your pockets?' With coat and trousers, I had many pockets. I put my hand in the rear pocket of my trousers and there they were. This pocket was normally used for my wallet, but I had put my wallet in an internal coat pocket for safekeeping.

'Oh hell, here they are,' I confessed, feeling like a complete dill.

Ian had his doubts about his cousin dating this uni student, but after getting over his great mirth he kindly said, 'Let's get back to the girls and tell them they had dropped down between the seats.' I was very grateful.

'Truth is Ian, I don't want her to go overseas. I might lose her.'

'Dennis, you're melodramatic. I think she's having some doubts. Let's see how it plays out.'

Kathy decided against her overseas trip, and I took it as part of her commitment to our relationship. Our love for each other grew from this point on.

****

She started coming to watch me play cricket, a game to which she had no prior interest. As the girlfriend of the captain, she happily took on the responsibility of doing the afternoon teas for the players. Kathy had just cleaned up the afternoon tea food, cups, and saucers and no sooner had come out to watch when she saw me felled whilst batting. I had been hit fair and square by a fast bowler in the 'goolies,' the 'crown jewels.' This was the second such experience of this nature. I failed to get the bat down in time, but I put everything behind the ball just as Uncle Ted had taught me. This time was worse than the schoolboy experience. The players lifted me to my feet and encircled me for privacy as I dropped my pants.

What greeted us was a ghastly sight, the plastic box had cracked and picked up a piece of my scrotum, and I was looking at a blood blister bubble of scrotum on the wrong side of the box. The look of amusement on the players who could see this turned to alarm, blood drained from their faces and they averted their eyes. All my blood was in the scrotal bubble. The umpire as well as the opposing captain broke the box open to release the squeezed scrotal skin. Two players walked me around the boundary line the long way. Well, they walked. I dragged my feet along as best I could. They hauled me to the club house and a waiting Kathy.

'Get the *Bird's Eye* onto them love,' one of the players told her as I was delivered into her care. This was all a bit embarrassing as we weren't even engaged yet. Kathy looked mystified.

'He means the frozen peas,' I interpreted.

'Oh, I see,' she hesitantly said.

I weakly replied, 'I hope you weren't expecting us to have any children.'

She blushed and said, 'Oh, Dennis. Don't joke about such things.'

45

DOWN THE PLATFORM I LOOKED

In the next long uni vacation of 1966/67, I was gaining work experience at an iron ore mine at Kooloonooka, Western Australia. The mine was run by the Western Mining Corporation, also known as WMC in the industry, a leading mining company of its day. My task was to conduct mapping on the southern extension of the ore body. It was excessively hot in the west.

My work with WMC was not unblemished. Somehow a party was in full process in my room at the demountable workers accommodation cabins. I didn't have the wherewithal to shut the party down. So, I became comprehensively drunk and at one point was outside on all fours in the dust looking a large dog in the eye, and he in turn licked me as though I was an ice cream. I did not have the power within me to brush the dog away. The dog lost interest when I heaved my guts out. Not even a dog wanted my company at that point. I was violently sick in my room and didn't make breakfast the next morning. Despite this, I was transported out to my mapping project by the Mine Site Geologist. Once he was out of sight, I scrambled beneath the shade of a tree with a water bottle to nurse my hangover and fell asleep. I was awoken shortly afterwards by the return of the geologist's car. The domestic staff had discovered the dreadful state of my room and rung the Mining Superintendent. The geologist returned me to my room via the pharmacist to collect some milk of magnesia and headache tablets with the instructions to clean the room, sleep it off, and to report to work the next morning.

The next morning was equally ugly as I was hauled in front of the Mining Superintendent and received a dressing down. 'You are a professional, or soon to be one. You should be ashamed of the state you were in and the state of your room. No one should be required to clean up such a mess after you. You are supposed to be an example to the workers. There will be no repetition of such behaviour. This incident will be going on your record.'

'Yes sir. It will not happen again.' I chastened.

'I should think not. Now get out of here and finish off that mapping. Only two weeks to go now I believe.'

'Yes, that's right.' I ruled a line through gaining future employment with WMC. I would like to say that that was the end of it, but there was one other incident on my last day. I had said my farewells to the Mining Superintendent and the geologist, I paid my outstanding bills, and then I found myself at the bar of the Kooloonooka Hotel waiting for the train to take me to Perth. I was surrounded by workers that I had befriended. I needed access to my room to get my luggage, and in doing so I was entrusted with a large bundle of keys for all the rooms in the camp. The wait for the train was longer than I had anticipated, and I was part of a group shouting rounds of drinks. The drinkers literally poured me onto the train. I dozed off and awoke when the train came to a halt at the siding of Perenjori. To my horror I discovered that I had the key ring containing all the keys to the camp cabins. What to do? I clambered from the train and raced up to the Station Master, explaining my plight. Could he get the keys back to Kooloonooka on the next train heading north? He assured me he could. Shaken, I returned to the train.

While at Kooloonooka, Kathy and I had exchanged romantic letters to each other. I still have the letters. I had made no mention of my indiscretions with drinking but, after too many drunken episodes, I had to admit that perhaps I had a problem with alcohol. I needed a strong woman to sort me out. Kathy could be just the one to mould me into a semi-respectable human being. I sobered up during the three-day trip on the train across the Nullarbor. It gave me a long time to reflect.

Absence does indeed make the heart grow fonder. I arrived back from WA by train to be greeted by both my parents and Kathy. My parents at this stage had not met Kathy and were somewhat surprised by the passion of our greeting. A deep kiss with Kathy, Marilyn Monroe like with her raising one lower leg in the air, seemed to unsettle them. A Tom Jones hit of the time was "*The Green Green Grass of Home.*" It contained the line, "*And down the road I looked and there runs Mary, hair of gold and lips like cherries.*" Well, Kathy ran down the platform with sun-tanned arms in a sleeveless, beautiful pale blue dress. I can remember it as though it was yesterday.

The twelve-week separation and the romantic letter exchange had made us hungry for each other. Each night for a fortnight we were not apart until university resumed. We had a whirlwind romance and were married in September 1967 with two thousand dollars to our name. It was all Kathy's money, so I can be accused of marrying for money. I was in my last year of university and penniless after buying the engagement ring. The one thing going for me was that I had a Commonwealth Scholarship. It provided a twenty dollar per week living allowance. Eighteen dollars of that went on rent. With the leftovers, we managed such wonderful staple meals as fifteen cent pot roasts. This involved rolled sausage meat roasted in the oven with vegetables. It sat very heavily. The meal could keep you going for days, especially with follow up slices of sausage meat and tomato sauce sandwiches. It must have helped me pass my degree as the weight of it kept me glued to a chair studying in the geology library.

We were from contrasting backgrounds, a WASP from the city and a Catholic country girl. When I announced that I was marrying a Catholic, I had cornered Dad around the incinerator in the backyard. This is where we Harrisons retreated to eat an orange. This was a dramatic contrast to Kathy's family as they tossed oranges around in their living room. They would peel them like an apple and slice the top third of them right through. With the rind intact, it was possible to eat the orange without a dripping mess. Wow, what an improvement.

Dad was shocked and most upset at the announcement.

'What's wrong with my boys?' he asked. 'Marrying a Catholic? My God, Grandfather will roll in his grave.' He violently poked some more garden clippings down into the incinerator, and smoke and ash spewed into the sky as he gazed into the depths of the bin. He added, 'I think you could have trouble becoming prime minister now, son.'

I am sure when we married many of our friends may have thought, *This will not last,* however our love for each other has been well tested, and stood those tests as we have celebrated our golden wedding anniversary. Dave was my best man and Trevor my groomsman, who else? Jill and Pam, Kathy's sister in law, were her bridesmaids.

****

Sometimes it is the smallest of things that you recall that represent a home. Dad, like many of his era, enjoyed playing practical jokes on the children in his life. I recall Uncle Alan and the sixpence in the glass. Dad's was to place a mixture of sugar coated and milk chocolate aniseed rings in a beautiful music box with a dancing ballerina figurine twirling in front of a mirror to the music of Swan Lake. He made sure that his grandchildren knew that there were sweets hidden in the music box, and so he had given specific instructions to ask Grandpa if they would like some. Then he would excuse himself and leave the room. Of course, it was a setup of temptation and the youngsters would inevitably try and surreptitiously steal one when Grandpa was not looking, only to be caught in the act because of the music. He loved that joke, and played it on Brian's children. And soon, eventually on my own.

The early departure from the family home of both Brian and me, both barely twenty-one years old, may have been influenced at a deep subliminal level due to the despair and hollowness of the family, Mum's cyclical illness, and Dad's head-in-the-sand response to her illness. They were independent acts and decisions of course, but we were each fleeing the mire of seemingly endless darkness into an open new dawn of possibilities.

****

I sat the last exam in the last week of November and started a job at the Victorian Mines Department the very next week. At last, our deficit budgeting could be turned around. The work at the Mines Department was anything but stimulating. Members of the public came in with their strange rocks and fossils, and I was given the task of identifying them. I looked around for alternatives. Employment was a necessity, Kathy was pregnant. Uncertain about the demands of field work and the lengthy periods away from home that it entailed, I applied for a Commonwealth cadetship to become a computer programmer. At the same time, I applied to be a geophysicist with Australian Aquitaine Petroleum (AAP), a subsidiary of the major French oil company Société Nationale des Pétroles d'Aquitaine (SNPA), now known as Elf Aquitaine.

'We have all the geophysicists we need right now, but we could offer you a position as a geologist,' the Aquitaine interviewer stated. 'The position is in Brisbane.'

'Could I respond to you next week after discussing this with my wife?' I replied.

I had been accepted in the computer programmer training cadetship which would have meant no field work and Melbourne domesticity. I was aware that one of the twenty graduates from our class of '67 switched to pharmacy as his fiancé refused to tolerate a life of separation due to the field work. Kathy could see the fire in my belly when I spoke of the opportunities in geology compared with working in the back room as a public servant on computer programs. We chose the expansive life of geology.

I had been living on my potential all these years. The potential of becoming, doing something significant. Becoming a good opening batsman, the encouragement of my father egging me on that one day I could become prime minister. Now was the time to deliver. I suppose Junior Petroleum Geologist with AAP was as good a start as any. My first day with Aquitaine was to be on the 19th of February, 1968. Something even bigger happened on the 20th February. It was then that I considered I entered adulthood.

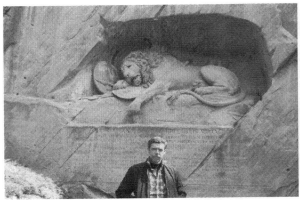

The Lion Monument Lucerne, Switzerland 1998

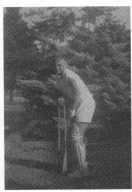

The Young Batsman, Floreat Park WA 1958

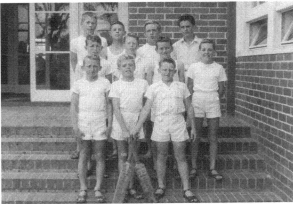

Captain Floreat Park Primary School Cricket Team, WA 1958

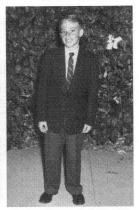

First Long Trousers, Perth WA 1959

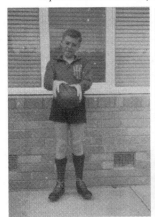

The Young Footballer, Elwood Victoria 1961

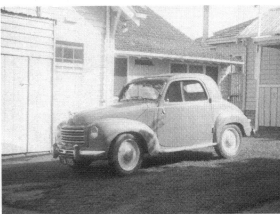

First Car Fiat 500 "Mighty Mouse", Glen Iris Victoria 1965

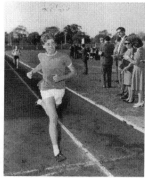

Winning the Elwood High School Mile 1963

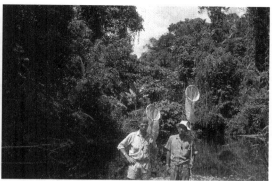

The Butterfly Catchers, New Guinea 1968

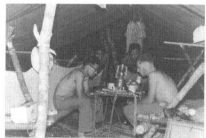

Playing Chess with Hero Under Canvas New Guinea, 1968

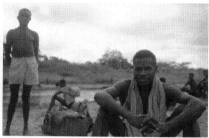

Carriers on river bend after my encounter with long-long native, New Guinea 1968

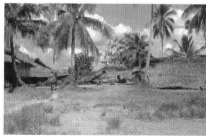

Native Village just before the Mutiny New Guinea 1968

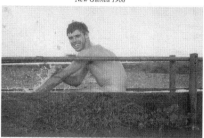

Sheep Trough Comes in Handy, WA 1968

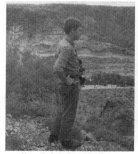

Young Geologist Examining Terrain Carnarvon Basin WA 1968

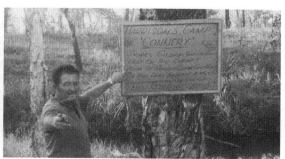

Harrison Camp Connery, Arnhem Land NT 1969

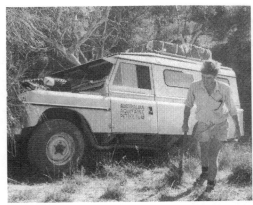

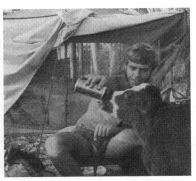

Camp Pet Receives a Drink Arnhem Land NT 1969

Arnhem Land was tough on Vehicles NT 1969

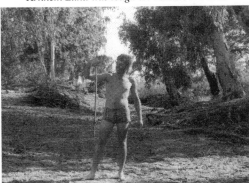

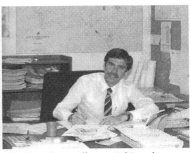

Chief Geologist Alliance Oil Development NL. Melbourne Vic 1982

One Dead Snake in Creek Bed Arnhem Land NT 1969

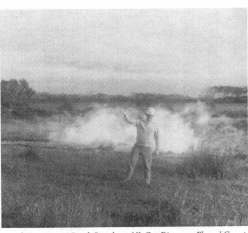

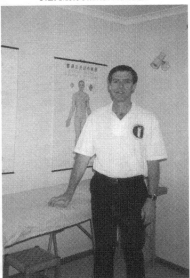

North Paaraate #1 Beach Petroleum NL Gas Discovery Flowed Gas at Rate of 7 MMcfd, near Timboon Victoria, 1979

Shiatsu and Chinese Masseuse, Carindale QLD 1996

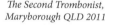

INVESTMENT

Financial Review, Wednesday, June 19, 1991

Crusader wins court dispute with Santos

By IAN HOWARTH

Oil and gas producer Crusader Ltd has won a major victory in its dispute with Santos Ltd over the operation of the Cooper Basin Gas Unit production agreement.

This means Crusader can reclaim more than $14 million paid under the altered terms of the agreement and raise its share of production revenue from the Cooper Basin gas project earned since 1987.

The Full Court of the SA Supreme Court yesterday overturned an earlier Supreme Court ruling in Santos favour.

The dispute arose following the January 1, 1987, review by Santos of the "participation factors" in the agreement.

Under the terms of the CBGU agreement, the participation factors are to be reviewed every two years.

The participation factors determine the percentage interest of each partner to the agreement in relation to project operating costs, revenue received and the percentage ownership in the event of one partner deciding to sell its stake in the gas project.

Santos, as project operator and the major interest holder, conducts the review, but must receive the unanimous agreement of each partner on the data used to calculate the new participation factors.

Crusader challenged the January 1987 review, but lost its initial court battle.

But on appeal, according to a Crusader statement last night, the Full Bench unanimously "found that the review and adjustment (of participation factors) had not been conducted by Santos in accordance with the unit agreement and was therefore not binding on any of the unit parties.

"The effect of the court's order is that Santos must re-prepare and re-submit the data upon which any review and adjustment of participation factors effective from January 1, 1987 is to be based.

"This data must be unanimously agreed by all of the participants or alternatively arbitrated ..."

The effect of yesterday's judgement is that:
- Crusader becomes entitled to repayment of money it had paid as a consequence of the 1987 review totalling about $14 million plus interest.
- Gas revenue participation factors are reinstated to the pre-January 1, 1987, level which results in Crusader's share increasing from the current 6.31 per cent to 8.29 per cent pending the completion of the new review.
- All parties to the Cooper Basin unit are reinstated to the positions they would have retained if the defective 1987 review had not occurred.

- Crusader was awarded costs of the appeal.

But the awarding of costs of the initial trial, totalling close to $2 million for each party, has not been settled.

Crusader's chairman, Mr Graham Tucker, said "the directors are pleased that the company's stance and that of its senior executives, on the conduct of the 1987 review and Adjustment by Santos has been vindicated by the court".

Santos said in a statement that it was currently considering its position following the appeal court judgement.

Santos has only two options. It can accept the decision of the Full Bench and rework the 1987 agreement, or it can take the matter to the High Court of Australia.

Most industry analysts contacted last night were sceptical about a High Court appeal.

Santos said that a recalculation of the 1987 participation factors "will not differ substantially from those originally calculated".

There are 11 participants to the original Cooper Basin gas unit agreement.

But four have subsequently been acquired by Santos leaving just Santos, Crusader, Delhi Petroleum (owned by Esso Australia), Sagasco Ltd, Bridge Oil Ltd and its subsidiary Bridge Oil Developments, and Basin Oil Ltd.

The Second Trombonist, Maryborough QLD 2011

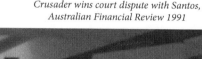

Crusader wins court dispute with Santos, Australian Financial Review 1991

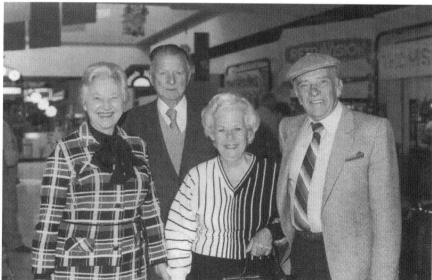

Mentors and family left to right – Aunty Joy, Uncle Ted, Mum, Dad, Perth WA 1986

PART 3 -
ADULTHOOD
1968 – 1991

"I write to gain meaning, interpret and understand. In shining a light on one of my struggles may it assist someone else's search"

Dennis Harrison

46

DENNIS HARRISON, WHO?

'Hello, it's Dennis Harrison here.'
'Who?'
'Dennis Harrison. I'm the junior geologist that started yesterday.'
'Oh yes.'
'Well, I can't come to work today, my wife's having a baby and the removalist is delivering our furniture.'
'I see. I'll tell Dr van der Welle.'
'Thank you.'

My uni mate, Frank Marsh, and I drove from Melbourne to Brisbane, thankfully not in the Fiat 500, but in my Aunt Joy's 1939 Vauxhall. I had bought it off her in one of those special family deals. Apart from the shorting out of the horn coming through Gundagai, the car had not missed a beat. Late in her pregnancy, Kathy decided to fly to Brisbane. Aquitaine had allowed us one week in a motel in order to find some permanent accommodation. We attempted the impossible, to buy a house in a week in a strange city. At the end of the week, we rented a flat opposite the Shafston Hotel in Wellington Rd, Kangaroo Point.

Aquitaine had put us up in the Coronation Motel on Coronation Drive in Milton. It was one of the best motels in Brisbane at the time, with a fabulous reputation for its seafood restaurant. We parked the 1939 Vauxhall amongst the Mercedes and Jaguars of the rich and famous, and within the week I had devoured the complete seafood menu and was coming back for seconds.

Due to Kathy's condition, and as I was beginning to realise the full responsibilities of adulthood, I did a dry run from the Coronation Drive to the Mater hospital. Just as well I did.

I commenced with AAP on Monday the 19th February 1968. I was so chuffed. I had landed a job and arrived in the big time after all those years of dedicated study. I said to Kathy, 'We've got to celebrate.' We went to Milano's, the leading restaurant in Brisbane at the time. Suitably satiated, we retreated to the Coronation Motel and put on the television to watch Hemingway's "*A Farewell to Arms.*"

As good as it was I did not see the film out, however, Kathy watched the whole thing. The character, Catherine, goes into labour and the delivery is exceptionally painful and complicated. Catherine delivers a stillborn baby and later dies of a haemorrhage. This was not the best movie for an expectant mother near term to view. Kathy was mortified. The next thing I knew, I was being shaken awake by Kathy. She was having contractions and thought it a good idea to go to the hospital. The strong Vauxhall bounced down Grey St, and I heroically delivered Kathy to the rear doors of the Mater. We were greeted by two nuns who took Kathy into their care. I was brusquely excused, getting the impression that this whole unfortunate episode was my entire fault. They might as well have said, 'Humph, men, they cause all the problems in this world.' Kathy and the nuns disappeared into the lift and the doors closed. I felt quite alone and out in the cold. No discussion back then of the husband being present at the birth.

****

Nicole was born at one minute past midday on the Tuesday. I had taken delivery of our effects and placed what minimal furniture we had in our flat. I went over to the Shafston Hotel and ordered a counter lunch; T-bone steak and a beer. After ordering I rang the hospital and asked, 'Has my wife Kathy had the child yet?'

'Just a moment, Mr Harrison. I think there is something happening right now,' was the reply. I was left dangling on the phone listening to the static as I sipped my beer. The T-bone arrived, and I nonchalantly selected a chip. After what seemed like an interminably long time, the nurse came back on the line to say, 'Your wife has just given birth. You have a daughter. Both your wife and daughter are fine.'

'Thanks so much,' I said. 'I'll be right over to see them.'

I hung up the phone and, reaching for another chip, I noticed that my hand was shaking. The chip floated in my oesophagus like tasteless cottonwool. The T-bone no longer had any appeal. I pushed the plate away and finished my beer. I was numb. I scanned the bar, they were all strangers and I had no friend with whom I could celebrate this amazing event.

****

I raced through the foyer of the Mater hospital in search of Kathy. On the way through, I purchased the Dr Spock book, "*Baby and Child Care.*" Over thirteen million copies sold worldwide, the cover proudly announced, so I figured that would have everything that Kathy would want to know about babies. I know she was tremendously grateful for the gift, but she may have liked the large bunch of flowers that Aquitaine sent the next day a lot better than the book. It was very nice of Aquitaine. I had only given them one day's work and they had put us up in a motel for a week and provided Kathy with those flowers. But still, I had so much potential. I had been told I could be prime minister one day.

47

DR GEERT VAN DER WELLE

I made it to work on my third day of employment, and so I started my grooming as a geologist. Everyone starting out in a career needs a good mentor. I was assigned to Dr Geert van der Welle, a soft rock specialist with a PhD in stratigraphy. As a junior geologist, most of my work was away from home and in the field. I had tried to prepare my wife years ago when I had "wooed" her with the romantic proposal, 'How would you like to be married to a geologist?' The first twelve years of my career involved intensive field work, and it meant that Kathy had to be extremely resourceful.

Eccentricity was the norm with the eclectic mix of scientists at Aquitaine and so many of them were French! Ah, but they had some of the best field camps of any exploration company then operating in Australia. Fine wine and French cuisine was to be enjoyed even when roughing it in the field. My mentor, Dr Geert van der Welle, was suitably eccentric. His responsibility was Australasian exploration outside of Australia, and he took me for an introductory two-week fieldwork trip to New Zealand. It was not arduous work as it involved hiring a car and examining road cuttings to understand the stratigraphy. It was not without its challenges though, and disturbing as Geert, after rounding curves, would forget to return to the left-hand side of the road. I would have to remind him constantly, 'Geert! Get left, quick! You're not in bloody Europe now.' Geert would stroke his moustache and mutter certain indecipherable French swear words before swerving back onto the correct side of the road. This was all done at remarkable speed. I had been a nervous passenger ever since my two accidents in my youth. I had experienced looking into the abyss with Dave.

The inevitable eventually happened. Geert was pulled over for speeding.

'Driver, can I see your driver's licence?' the officer demanded.

Geert handed him his licence. 'Dutch. I see,' the policeman remarked.

Geert replied, 'Yes officer, I am a Dutchman working for a French oil company based in Australia, doing a little project in New Zealand,' and pointing to the licence whilst stroking and brushing his moustache said, 'That's my New Guinea's drivers licence.'

This was all too much for the local policeman, and he folded the licence back and returned it to Geert with the words, 'Well when in New Zealand just drive to the speed limits would you? Take care Doctor, and get on your way.'

Geert carefully drove away and stopped shortly after at a roadside café for a short black coffee. He lit up a filter-less, Gitane Brun; the classic, strong, French cigarette with the distinctive aroma, like dried camel dung had been rolled with the dark tobacco leaves.

Until the French government imposed levies on cigarettes they were relatively cheap, and they helped define the classic, exciting Frenchman image, complete with the aura of sexuality defined by the gypsy woman playing the tambourine on the packet cover. What was the way he stroked and brushed his moustache all about? It was like a preening; he'd flick it up with his index finger and then brush it down again. It was presumably vanity, image, and habit. I was learning. I hadn't thought about image much up until this point in my life. I had tried, quite unsuccessfully, the professorial look of smoking a pipe while at university. I gave that up as I clamped on the pipe stem so hard that it was affecting my back molars and giving me lockjaw. I had decided that comfort and health were more important than image. Maybe suitable props to hide behind would be discovered later in life.

'You were bloody lucky back there, Geert,' I proffered, 'Liked the way you handled the cop though.'

Geert delayed his response for a moment taking a long draw on his Gitane, ejected a spiral of smoke and then responded, 'The lesson my boy is, everything is negotiable. Thinking on your feet, adaptability means survival. Enough of New Zealand Dennis. Next New Guinea, ha!'

'I can't wait, Geert,' I answered. The trouble was I hadn't yet broken the news to Kathy that I would be facing six months of field work in New Guinea with only a fortnight break back in AAP's Brisbane office.

****

In the fortnight after the New Zealand trip, Kathy came down with mastitis, also known as milk fever. As I was hanging Nicole's nappies on the community clothes line I was approached by the big Norwegian landlord of the Shafston flats. I related Kathy's problem to him. He was most sympathetic and in his slow broken English told me, 'Oh, very sorry. That is very serious in cows.' I understood it was very painful for Kathy.

Kathy is a very strong, stoic, and independent woman. Here she was alone in Brisbane with her first baby and no family or friends, all of whom were in Melbourne. She had befriended Elaine in the flat above ours. When I was in New Zealand, Kathy experienced her first of the tropical electrical storms that hit Brisbane during the summer months. Elaine, knowing that Kathy would be terrified, joined Kathy in our flat to comfort her until the storm was over. Elaine was now helping Kathy through the mastitis illness, but her assistance was limited as she had her own child to look after. We sent out an SOS to the family down south.

The fittest member of both our families at the time was Kathy's grandma. In later years, for the purposes of our children, we referred to her as 'big grandma' to distinguish her from Kathy's mum who was simply 'grandma.' She was seventy-eight years old and walked with a crutch for stability. I picked her up at the airport and she strode to my car with great purpose. She was here to save her beloved granddaughter from this madman named Dennis that had taken her away from Melbourne. Being wanted had given her a new lease of life. She took control of the house while Kathy was recovering. She would tuck Nicole under her arm and carry her from room to room, cook meals, clean and iron. She was a powerhouse.

She thought Kathy should have married a public servant, somebody in the Post Office or the Railways, maybe even a banker. Anyone other than a geologist. What was a geologist anyway? Nobody knew what a geologist did, including me so early on in my career.

Big grandma and I never agreed on politics, but I did feel very close to her. She had wonderful qualities and her strength flowed from her to her daughter and her granddaughter. They all ultimately accepted the fact that this renegade had entered their midst.

48

ON ASSIGNMENT IN WEWAK, NEW GUINEA

Opportunity and growth comes from the unique circumstances that individuals are placed in and the people to whom, and experiences to which, they are exposed. Life was whirling ahead at an unsustainable pace, and I was fortunate to have joined the international petroleum company, Aquitaine. It was one of the few companies still doing their own raw regional mapping.

I flew into Wewak, a town on the shores of Northern New Guinea, on the 31st of May, 1968, together with Geert who was the AAP team leader in charge of the exploration program. The heady smell of Geert's *Gitanes* added to the romance and excitement.

The Wewak airstrip was built by the Japanese and bombed by the Americans in World War II. The Wom Peninsula juts out into the Bismark Sea with beautiful white coral beaches backed by coconut palms. There is the shock of in-your-face colour. Rich tropical green contrasts with all the shades of blue as the ocean gently shelves towards land.

Geert broke into my observations, 'See those holes down there alongside the airstrip full of water?'

'Oh, yes.'

'They are the remains of bomb craters when the Allies drove the Japanese off the island in WWII. Wewak was the location of the Japanese surrender of this area. There is a memorial on the Wom Peninsula commemorating the event. By the way I don't have to remind you do I but don't mention the war to Yoshi and Hiroshi. Very sensitive you know,' Geert said as he bristled his moustache. The New Guinea exercise was a joint venture with the national

Japanese oil company, Japex, with AAP being the senior party and operator of the exploration licence.

The Douglas DC3 touched down on the tarmac with a jolt and the whole plane shuddered as the props went into reverse. The plane taxied to the fabricated building called the Wewak airport. As the doors opened the hot steamy air entered the plane carrying with it a complex mix of rich, musty tropical aromas. Once inhaled, never forgotten. There to meet us was Philippe Despres and two New Guinea boys, Winchet and Baro. Philippe was all action, one of the world's true hustlers. Most of the time language was not a handicap, what could not be understood could be adequately communicated with an array of gestures and arm waving.

'Allez, allez boys, the luggage… Hurry to the green machine,' he said as he hustled the local boys along. The green machine was a battered old land-rover that had seen its best days during the Second World War. I thought it just as well that Philippe had been a mechanic. He had been with AAP for over twenty years in the capacity of mechanic, cook, and field camp manager. Right now, he was in control of the Wewak base camp and provided key supplies and logistics support to the geologists.

'Allez, allez,' he repeated. 'Merde, this is not Sunday.' I looked around wondering what the urgency was; there were no traffic jams in Wewak. The locals languidly sauntered around either on foot or by bicycle, interspersed with some motorbikes and even fewer cars and trucks. It was just Philippe's nature. In his mind, things only got done when there was the appropriate level of drama, urgency, and excitement no matter how trivial the task. Much like my father really. This approach had got Philippe through to his pre-retirement years, so why change now? He was short with a well-developed paunch, bald-headed with two strips of tightly trimmed grey hair on both sides of the bald central strip. He was a bundle of fitness and energy and had that southern European skin that tans so well.

It was a short drive to the base camp, which consisted of two Besser-brick concrete buildings each with tanks at the rear catching water off the corrugated iron roofs. They had been rented off the Catholic mission. The Catholic mission had built a number of these dwellings for local housing, but in the short term welcomed the rental income provided by Aquitaine during their field season. They were of simple construction and design with six bedrooms off a central corridor and a kitchen down the rear of the building. One of the houses was used for accommodation and the other for an office.

Already in residence at the base camp were Yoshi and Hero and another Australian AAP geologist, Ray. Geert and Yoshi warmly greeted each other as they had spent several field seasons together on this project. They had obviously developed a great friendship. Hero and I were the new kids on the block and would require some training as to program execution. With a previous year's field season under his belt, Ray was regarded as experienced, now a senior. Ray had advised me back in the Brisbane office how to prepare for the New Guinea field work.

'The geology's one thing; learn as much Pidgin English as you can before you go. To help pass the time we all collect butterflies and native art,' Ray advised. 'The Sepik art is some of the best in the Pacific.' So, I had armed myself with Pidgin English and French–English dictionaries and a butterfly book, together with the necessary equipment for butterfly collection.

It was now late afternoon. We were assigned our bedrooms and Philippe disappeared to prepare the evening welcoming dinner. I had been told that he was a great cook and he never disappointed. *Steak Diane*, macaroni cheese, onions, and some unknown native greens for mains, followed by a cheese platter all washed down by a fine McWilliams Shiraz. The talk around the table quickly focussed on the political turmoil in France. Geert and Philippe in the main spoke in English but would occasionally break out into French when excited.

'It was initially only a small minority of students at *Université de Nanterre*. They were all followers of the Mao Tse Tung form of communism. That's what caused it!' Geert said.

'And now it has spread to the Sorbonne and dragging in other universities,' replied Philippe. 'There are now over twenty thousand students protesting. *Merde, les étudiante sont enragé, long-long.*' He was getting excited, animatedly waving his arms, and now mixing

English, French, and Pidgin English words. It was hard for me to keep up with the conversation and impossible to participate.

'De Gaulle's fled the country. Pompidou didn't know where *La Présidente* was for over six hours. He showed up in Germany.'

'*Il est un désastre.*'

'What's so surprising it's frozen France – the borders are closed because customs are closed. There is no petrol moving around the country. Il est tumult.'

'*Merde, les étudiante sont juste hors de couche.*' (trans: just out of nappies)

'If the Communists get into power the franc will be worthless. Aquitaine will feel the pinch.'

'We might have to emigrate to Australia permanently Philippe, what do you say?' Geert asked before continuing 'Australia is the best country. You know Australia should develop its beef industry. This is the growth industry – best beef in the world.'

This was the party breaker comment as we all thanked Philippe for the wonderful Steak Diane, and Geert closed with, 'Let's meet after breakfast to discuss the program. *Bonne soir messieurs.*'

****

At breakfast, Philippe introduced me to the red fleshed New Guinea pawpaw.

'Here, squeeze some lemon juice over it,' he advised.

'This is terrific Philippe, exquisite,' I commented. I still had the voracious appetite of youth. I would have the distinction to be the only AAP employee to ever put on weight during a New Guinea field season due to the over consumption of Tom Piper tinned puddings and condensed cream when out in the field.

We gathered in the office after breakfast.

'Messieurs, if this sounds like Geology 101, I apologise in advance, but it is important that we all understand the program requirements. In the three previous field seasons, we have defined the stratigraphic sequence. This season is all about structure. We are looking for something to drill. We already have some early indications at Nambilo and Mia Mia so we need to detail those structures and we need to cover the acreage to see if there are more to be found. We will be working principally south of the Bewani and Toricelli Ranges, heading towards the Sepik Valley,' Geert stated as he extended his *Gitane* loaded forefinger towards the map, bristling his moustache with the other forefinger. 'Not much outcrop to observe once you get onto the Sepik floodplain of course, so we will mostly work the foothills of the ranges.'

'Hero and Dennis, you both have to learn how we actually get around in the field. I have talked it over with Yoshi and we believe that we need a two day shake down trip near Maprik. Yoshi will take Hero as one party and Ray, you'll take Dennis and train him up as the other party. We can drive to Maprik and stay in the Maprik Hotel overnight, then head off the next day. I'll be staying in Wewak for discussions with our adjacent permit holders, Continental.'

'*Ils sont trop d'arbre sur le montée*, so no outcrops there. The outcrop is all in the creeks and rivers. Ray, show Dennis and Hero a page out of your field book from last year,' Geert instructed.

Ray dutifully passed Geert his field book.

Geert opened the book, selected a page, and continued, 'See, this is the idea. You walk the creek or river taking compass readings and make an estimate of the distance of the river as a series of straight line segments, and then plot it on the graph paper. Record your observations against the river sketch. When you get back to Wewak actual locations of the observations are then transferred on to the aerial photographs. We don't take the photographs into the field as they just get ruined.'

'I want you to concentrate on good in *situ* strike and dip readings, record any faults, and be observant for any salt water seeps or indications of oil, whether it be seep or scum or maybe stranded bitumen. '*Hommes, vous sommes nous yeux et oreilles*.' (trans: Men, you are our eyes and ears)

'We need a few organisational days in the base camp here before we set off to find all that oil. Yoshi and Ray, see if you can instruct *les nouveux garçons* as to how to prepare for a field trip. Once you have shown them that and how to calculate food requirements, Philippe, I suggest you take Hero and Dennis into town for general shopping. We will need two or three days here in Wewak to organise aerial photos and supplies. This will be some of the best days of your life lads, enjoy but be diligent.' And with an exhalation of smoke from the chain smoking Geert, we were dismissed.

49

SNAKE! SNAKE! SNAKE!

The shakedown trip near Maprik was not my finest hour. It must have crossed Geert's mind that I be returned to desk duties in Brisbane. After the return to base camp, I had come down with a severe case of dysentery. They had not warned me about drinking straight from the creeks. It is recommended to boil water each night when setting base camp and transfer that boiled water to your water flasks overnight for the next day. Ray had not taught me that lesson in time. Geert taught me one of his tricks which was to add a little red wine to the flask to make a weak wine cordial. It is most refreshing.

It was what happened on the trip, rather than after the trip, that caused Geert's moustache to bristle. My first night under canvas was a nightmare both for me and Ray. The field work modus operandi was for the geologist to fly into a village with a native boss boy and cook boy, and hire a team of native boys as carriers (in those days, the accepted term for the locals who assisted us was 'native' and 'boy.' It is no longer the case and inappropriate, however I use the terms here in order to be authentic to the time period). The number of carriers was determined by the planned number of days of field mapping, which ranged from one week to two weeks, averaging ten days. The geologist and the boss boy carried no cargo. The first calculation was to determine how many carriers were required to carry two tarpaulins, cooking utensils, food, and personal effects for the geologist. The next calculation was to determine how many carriers were required to carry the first tranche of carriers' food. This was followed by how many carriers were required to carry the second tranche of carrier food. The calculation was conducted to a converging end point. For the shakedown trip, we had driven to Maprik and for a two-man, two-day trip, the operating party was quite small.

Ray showed me how to walk the creeks with your geology boy. The geology boy carried a backpack that contained your G-Pick (also known as a geology hammer), your lunch, and any samples that you might collect. The geologist only carried a hard covered A5 sized notebook that had gridded graph paper, a clinometer (for measuring the dip and strike of the rocks), and a compass. The creek traverse was sketched, and observations entered in the notebook.

Overnight camp was under a tarpaulin. The tropical timber is so soft that the natives in quick time would cut down tree branches with a machete to make a ridge pole and two tent poles. These were lashed together by strips of native grass or stripped bark, depending upon what was available. Guy ropes were attached to the sides of the tarpaulin. The natives would construct a bed consisting of two poles inserted into a canvas sleeve braced on either end by crossed over poles laced together by the native 'rope.' Over the bed was a light framed structure to secure the mosquito net, a necessary preventative against malaria. In addition, they made a table upon which to eat and write up field notes.

The natives constructed a camp for themselves downstream from the geologist's camp. Camp construction could take up to an hour and was the most active time for the carriers. The boss boy controlled the team of carriers and during the day, they would make their own pace down the creek and have adequate rests putting their cargo down at bends in the river. The geologist, while working, would walk only with the geology boy.

Camp would be broken early morning after breakfast, and walking might commence by seven am and would conclude at three o'clock in the afternoon. While the natives were constructing the camp was a good time for the geologist to take a swim and a wash in the creek.

All this information had nothing to do with geology but everything to do with logistics and survival. It was a long way away from the geology library at Melbourne University, which had been my preparation.

So, here I was under canvas after my first day of operational training. Ray was not an easy character to like. He had a superior know-it-all attitude, a sense of humour to which I could not relate, and a loose dedication to the task at hand. The bottom line was he either didn't want to be a geologist or he wasn't looking forward to his second field season in New Guinea. For him, it seemed to be only an opportunity of purchasing some more Sepik art. The natives had set up our two beds under the fly tarpaulin with a table in between for our evening meal. Ray and I consumed our bowl of rice and tinned curried chicken, had a chat about the day, and then went straight to sleep.

I woke in the middle of the night in a lather of perspiration, yelling, 'Snake, snake!' I was fighting it off my leg, tangled up in this damned mosquito net. Ray had jumped out of his bed and shone his torch at me. I yanked the net off its flimsy frame and ran my arms up and down my legs in an attempt to brush off the snake.

'Are you alright? Are you alright?' he fearfully asked.

'I think so,' I replied.

'Where's the snake?'

'It must have gone.'

'Bloody hell. How big was it?'

'Thick as my wrist. Must have been a python, maybe a carpet snake I guess. I didn't see it, just felt it on my leg,' I explained.

'Jesus. My first thought was you were being attacked by a native. Let's have some of that cold tea and then get back to sleep,' Ray said.

It wasn't until the next morning that I had the courage to tell him what had happened. It was a nightmare, induced by sleeping on my arm that had 'gone to sleep,' draped as it was across the pole that was within the canvas sleeve of the bed. The arm had become a dead weight. When I was rolling over in the bed the deadened arm had flopped onto my leg, and I had grabbed it with my other arm believing it to be a snake, which is why I had started fighting with it. There was no snake. I was fighting with my arm. The incident may have induced Ray's early exit from geology when he returned to Brisbane.

The cook boy was very slow coming up from the carrier's camp the next morning. I saw his round face and fearful brown eyes appear from behind a tree.

'Master,' he whispered to Ray. 'Is everything okay?'

'Yes, Baro.'

'We heard these screams in the middle of the night. We thought the evil spirit, Masalai belong riva, come up and get one of you.'

'No, Baro. We're okay. Dennis had a nightmare. He thought he was fighting a snake in his bed.'

'Ah, so good, so good. Very happy he okay. What you have for breakfast?'

'I'll have my normal, tea and some rice left over from last night. What about you Dennis?'

'Ah, yes tea and some of that corned beef on Saos.'

'You'll soon get over that stuff,' Ray laughed.

50

LOOKING INTO THE ABYSS AGAIN

Now fully trained to the wiles of New Guinea, I was to lead my own team. Geert assigned Baro, the experienced cook, and Paos, a new boss boy, to me.

'Dennis, vous sommes nous yeux et oreilles,' he told me as he pointed two fingers towards his eyes, then at me. 'Look out for yourself and no more nightmares.'

'There'll be no more repeats of that, Geert,' I said.

'How many carriers do you need for this first trip?'

'Fifteen.'

'Right, well ring ahead to the Catholic mission in Dreikikir and let the priest know. He will line up the boys for when you fly in.'

On this trip I was flying in and out of Dreikikir conducting river traverses both north and south with a ridge traverse back to where I had started. This was unusual. It was more normal to fly into one village and then out of another. Dreikikir is quite a famous airstrip in New Guinea with a church at one end and a hospital at the other. The plane landed uphill on the grassy strip and taxied to the top of the slope, where passengers and cargo were unloaded. That was relatively painless and enjoyable. Take off, however, was far more disturbing. The single engine Dornier would furiously vibrate with cargo rattling as the pilot maxed out the throttle. He would then release the brake and hurtle the plane full bore down hill, take the dog leg to the left, pull back on the control stick, and no sooner had the plane become airborne, would have to bank to the right to miss the church steeple at the bottom of the runway. More excitement than the big dipper at Luna Park, and it encouraged everyone to cross themselves regardless of belief or non-belief. Being so close to a hospital provided little comfort.

The areas assigned to me for mapping were dominated by villages controlled by Catholic missions. They flew the single engine Dornier Do27 planes. Their Protestant competitors were the Missionary Aviation Fellowship (MAF) who had a fleet of single engine Cessna 185's. No matter how carefully Paos selected our team of carriers, we would inevitably end up with one or two that were not up to the task because of some injury or illness. I was the default medical officer and at the end of each day would treat minor and not so minor injuries. The worst sights were some of the tropical ulcers that were treated with sulphonamide powder and antibiotics. It was common to see many natives with the skin disease 'Kas Kas,' a type of scabies caused by a parasitic mite, resulting in unpleasant looking and dry, flaky skin runs. Paos was afflicted by this.

The biggest danger of course was catching malaria. We all took Chloroquine tablets religiously every Sunday. They turned your skin yellow. I continued taking the tablets for an extra month after returning from the second and final three-month assignment, but I still contracted malaria. I had seen enough of it in New Guinea to know all the symptoms. I had the common Vivax malaria, which involved a twenty-four-hour cycle of being relatively well one day but struck down the next with a fever and the shakes. It took me a week to convince a southern doctor that I had malaria. He eventually conceded, and finally I was admitted to hospital to be treated with Primaquine. Thankfully, the treatment eradicated the parasite from my liver and I have never had a recurrence. Because of this experience I believe that Chloroquine is only a suppressant and not an absolute preventative.

I had seen the dramatic effects of malaria. I was traversing a long straight stretch of river with my geology boy when in the distance I saw a native, well ahead, enter the water and commence walking towards me. Even from a distance there appeared to be something strange about this fellow. I was alert to all possibilities. I decided to walk to one bank of the river and he walked to the same bank. I transferred to the other side of the river and he followed. This fellow wanted a confrontation or a meeting at the very least. We zigzagged towards each other until we were face to face. Thankfully, he carried no obvious weapons on him. His eyes looked crazed, his body frame shook, and he did not look to be in control of his limbs. He did however move very swiftly, and he grabbed my notebook from my hands and started turning the pages, stabbing them wildly while alternatively looking at me and then the notebook. He spoke some insane guttural gibberish whilst stabbing the book. I lost my composure and snatched the book back and started walking away, leaving him stranded in the river.

The team of carriers were waiting ahead on the next curve in the river having a rest and had seen it all. They were in hysterics, they thought the whole thing had been very amusing.

'What's so funny, boys?' I asked.

'Master, him-ee long long,' Paos explained to me as he made small circles with his index finger around his ear.

'What you mean?'

'He's got malaria.'

'Oh, I did not know,' I replied. I looked back down the river, but he had disappeared. I subsequently understood the dreadful effects of cerebral malaria leading to insanity and ultimate death.

****

On another trip I was seated under a native hut. Through Paos, I had asked if there was any native art in the village that I could see and maybe purchase. There was much activity amongst the villagers, and I was surrounded by people. It was some time before my attention was drawn to their feet. Many had the deformed feet of leprosy, swollen feet with fused toes retreating into a formless foot. Not understanding the disease or the risks it may have presented, I thanked them for their time and retreated to the river to set up camp for the night and take a much-needed bathe.

I had the good fortune to meet a Catholic priest who was in charge of the leprosarium at Aitape. He was a charming man, a good conversationalist, and enjoyed a nip of Warrior dark rum, a New Guinea concoction. His dedication to the welfare of the natives and the passion with which he explained his service to them impressed me. He had worked in leper colonies in both Tibet and China up until 1952. He then came to Aitape to continue his work. In 1952 Mao Tse Tung required all missionaries to leave China. I told him of the village I had come across that had many lepers. He thanked me for the information and said that he would go to the village to encourage them to go to Aitape for treatment.

'How far west are you penetrating with your geology surveys?' the priest asked while we were sharing our tot of rum.

'So far, Tila is the most west I have made.'

'Some of the natives that have come to the leprosarium have reported that there are tribes west of Tila, towards the headwaters of the Sepik River on the West Irian border, who still practice cannibalism.'

'You have to be joking,' I scoffed.

'No. You should be aware that for some of the natives you meet on your surveys it will be the first time they will have seen or met a white man.'

"Hell,' I said. 'Give me another slug of that rum, Father.'

****

Apart from the demanding take off from the Dreikikir airstrip, I experienced many disconcerting flights. The two that I recall most readily were while flying with the MAF. The first incident was on a long return flight from Tila in the West Sepik to Wewak and, whether it was due to the plane carrying excess cargo or pilot miscalculation, we were running short of fuel. Flying low with the beautiful shoreline of Wewak in sight, the pilot was alternatively tipping the plane from one side to the other to allow whatever fuel was still contained within the wing fuel tanks to flow to the engine.

As serious as this incident was, it pales into insignificance when compared with the second experience. I was returning with the MAF from a field trip that required us to put down at Lumi to pick up two native missionaries. They were to be taken to the village of Anguganak to attend a Brethren conference. (The Brethren are a New Zealand sect serviced by the MAF). We dropped them off, refuelled, and then took off for Wewak which was approximately one hundred and ninety kilometres east north east from Anguganak.

The route would require us to fly over the coastal Toricelli Ranges. We went straight into an electrical storm. I was seated in the cockpit alongside the pilot. The thunderous rain pounded against the window of the plane. There was zero visibility. We were flying purely on the instruments and I knew we had to ascend to get over the mountains. The plane was being buffeted from side to side and would rise and fall quickly in altitude. The pelting rain made such noise that I couldn't communicate with the pilot. All I could do was look at the compass and I saw that we were heading north east and then north. I would steal sideways glances at him to determine if he knew what he was doing and that he was in command of the situation.

My one control on my future rested with my watch and the compass readings. If I could survive a crash into the jungle maybe I could have a rough concept of location through an understanding of flight time and direction. Merde, now we were heading northwest and then west. When I observed the compass reading south I was convinced that I was cactus.

We broke out of the dense blackness and, with rain reduced to mere hard rather than pelting, I sighted an airstrip below. The pilot indicated to me with a thumbs-up that we were going to land on the strip. He made a perfect landing and taxied to the shed at the end of the strip.

I sat numb in the cockpit, still surrounded by too much noise to talk to the pilot. When he turned the engine off he said, 'I couldn't find a hole in the storm so after a while I decided to return to Anguganak on the instruments.'

'Bloody well done. Thank goodness you did,' I said.

'We'll be here for the night, and try for Wewak in the morning, weather permitting.'

'Sounds good to me.' I felt like kissing the guy or the airstrip itself when I stepped out from the plane, much like the Pope when he lands on a new continent. We had flown in one big circle for over an hour. We joined the Brethren for a simple dinner and after dinner gathering. I joined them in singing their hymns with great vigour and thanksgiving that evening.

****

The recovery time in Wewak was spent writing up our field notes and revising our maps, treating any blistered feet and wounds, as well as making preparations for the next mission. Even when in Wewak it wasn't without excitement. We experienced some heavy earthquakes. I was awoken one evening to the sloshing sound of water as it was being thrown from one side to the other in the tanks at the rear of our dwelling. My bed was moving backwards and forwards. Ornaments and books were being thrown from the shelves, and I pulled the pillow over my head. When the worst of it seemed to be over, I raced for the door but I couldn't get out as the door had jammed in the distorted frame. At one lucky break in the cycle of vibrations, the door freed and I raced out the central corridor to the rear of the dwelling. Philippe, Ray, and Hero were already in the backyard. The fear was palpable and expressed in their eyes.

I was at the Wewak airport when the 'big daddy' climax of this series of earthquakes that had persisted for about a fortnight hit. I was inside a hangar some four metres in height that had triangulated steel uprights and roof trusses. I saw the uprights wave like a hula dancer's hips, and a wave move through the bitumen runway. We aborted any flight from Wewak that day. On exiting the road back to our accommodation, there was a crack in the road that you could fit your whole hand down. Walking the creeks and rivers in the field showed plenty of evidence of the effects of earthquakes. Big landslides are seen where rocks, soil, and trees come away leaving massive scars and block the valleys. Water is banked back behind these landslides. This can cause villages to be flooded upstream of the blockage and, if it is breached or broken, can cause serious flooding to the villages downstream.

With massive tropical rainfall, streams and rivers can rise and fall very quickly. This was something to which we had to be aware on our field traverses and the setting of our overnight field camps.

51
MUTINY ON THE SEPIK

'Beware the armchair general' was one of the lessons of Gallipoli. At the tender age of twenty-two, and not sufficiently well read, I did not yet understand the lesson.

We were coming to the end of our field season and Geert was about to fly in to review our progress and shut down the operation. We had been given an expected termination date of October 14th. Ray, Hero, and I had some detailing to do on the Saran anticline, a potential target, and had designed a creative, if not ambitious, program.

The plan was for me to fly into Lumi with Baro, my cook boy, and the two boss boys Paos and Winchet, hire a big team of forty carriers, and walk them to the village of Abrau, thirty-five kilometres to the south. It was anticipated that the remote Abrau would not be capable of supplying that many carriers. Ray and Hero were to fly into Abrau and utilise twenty-six natives for one survey and I would use fourteen for my separate survey. This was a large operation, and two planes were required to fly the cargo into Lumi. We had agreed that I needed three days to walk such a large crew from Lumi to Abrau. We had allocated a full day just to assemble the forty men.

Our illustrious leader Geert flew in and thought this was far too generous, and that I could complete the walk to Abrau in two days. We conceded, but it was a mistake. It was impossible to keep such a large group moving together despite the efforts of both Paos and Winchet. The walking was difficult up and down the steep hills and valleys, and the boys were carrying heavy sixty-pound packs. I pushed them hard the first day, and by nightfall we were not even half way. The second day was even harder than the first and upon arriving at a village still north of Abrau, I was facing a mutiny. Half my carriers quit. They dropped their cargo and refused to proceed. I left Winchet and ten boys with cargo in the village, and then pushed on to Abrau with Baro, Paos, and ten boys. Baro and I arrived at Abrau at six thirty in the evening. Paos and his depleted team joined us at eight o'clock. We were all exhausted. So much for Geert's adjusted planning. I had walked the boys into the ground and they would be broken carriers for the rest of the mission.

Hero had flown in alone at five o'clock. Ray had come down with malaria and, in the Wewak hospital, was incapable of making the trip. We had to rest the carriers the next day while Paos and Baro visited the surrounding villages to recruit new ones. Hero and I redesigned the survey programs.

Just as Kenny Rogers sings in the *"The Gambler"* - *'You've got to know when to hold 'em and know when to fold 'em;'* this was a salutary lesson in backing your own judgement in life.

****

I was to return the following year with Geert to conduct some sampling. The sole purpose of our return was to determine the important porosity and permeability values of our reservoir rocks through the collection of suitable samples. We flew into our target area by helicopter then dropped into a river bed from which we would be picked up the same day. We were armed with jam tins with lids. The sediments were so young that we had initially thought we could simply push or lightly tap the tin with a hammer into the rock face.

We walked the river stopping at suitable outcrops with an entourage of inquisitive natives in tow. We would talk to them and share with them our cigarettes, chocolate and odd sweets. They loved tobacco and would smoke just about any dry leaf that they could find.

The rocks proved to be too solid for our sampling technique, so we would have to break a large piece off with the hammer and then fashion a cylinder of rock that would fit into the can using a knife. We hammed it up for the natives and pretended to eat the rock saying, 'Himee good pela kai kai.' The natives thought this was hilarious.

Finally, the helicopter arrived to whisk us away. No doubt such an experience to the many natives was amazing and supported the cargo cult mentality of the Pacific. The stories told by them back in their villages would have been too wild for many to believe, 'They were rock eaters I tell you!'

52

UNDER DURESS SCIENCE OF NO HELP

Within 12 months I had been transformed from a university student to a man with a wife and daughter catching butterflies, walking creeks, and mixing with lepers in New Guinea. How was my mind to process all of this?

Confronted with so much danger - earthquakes, malaria, dysentery, skin diseases, knowing the incidents of plane and helicopter crashes, living with the indigenous people that might turn on you, going into areas in which you are the first white man many of them have ever seen, and knowing that some cannibalism was still present in tribes near the West Irian border in the West Sepik province... all of this led me to examine my own mortality, the fragility and impermanence of life. Seeing the dedication and strength of the Catholic priests and nuns who devoted their lives selflessly to improving the lives of the natives moved me in ways that I could not yet understand. But when you have seen and experienced these things, they are never forgotten. They permanently reside in your psyche. You have walked the walk. Trudging up the creeks and rivers, slipping on the boulders, sinking in sand up to your waist hoping like hell you can extract your foot and it doesn't suck you in any further, wading waist deep in water with a snake swimming towards you; it is possible you might just blink, think and understand this is humanity, this is life, and death may be close, unsighted, but around the corner. It was then, in an attempt to find meaning, that I started to look for answers in religion. If life is confronted and confronted fully, the risks fully understood, then perhaps more people would actively seek religion out to find meaning. If, however, it is lived out in the comfort of western first world experiences, sipping lattes and eating donuts, unaware of the labour and suffering that goes behind the production of the consumer products that are being enjoyed, perhaps then you can live without religion, but then it becomes a gutted, empty life, does it not? One divorced from real life lived in an artificial void.

Agnostics would argue it is they that understand reality, and that the religious have constructed an artificial God. However, the irreligious have intellectualised and theorised a cerebral existence of equal fantasy, another construct the pillars of which are unproven. Many divorced from the understanding of the power of nature throughout the millennia (the evidence of which is in the rock record) may believe that man has control over climate. If they only knew the levels of uncertainty contained within this magnificent Earth of ours they would understand the shaky pillars upon which that premise, modelling, and belief stands.

53

THE PANHANDLE SETS IN THE WEST

In 1969 Kathy and I bought our first house in Jindalee, a western suburb of Brisbane, for twelve thousand dollars. We were to sell it two years later for fourteen thousand dollars in one of my less brilliant career moves when we went to an iron ore mine in the Northern Territory.

Perhaps of bigger moment; in 1969 AAP's Petrel No 1 well blew out in the Bonaparte Gulf and it took fourteen months to bring it under control. The damaged rig was towed to Singapore for repairs. Fourteen months later, it returned to drill the relief well, Petrel 1A, which involved a horizontal drilled section to intersect with the original blow out zone, down which cement was poured. Before the killing of the Petrel blow out, I flew over the big turbulent gas bubble on the surface of the ocean on my way for well site training on Gull No. 1.

The blow out was a major setback on petroleum operations for the company, and I was transferred during the year to conduct some mineral search field work in Arnhem Land. It involved a demanding twelve weeks away from Kathy and Nicole. Aquitaine's mineral search was driven by the SNPA academic Pierre Nicolini who had concocted a scientific theory and wrote a book entitled "*Gîtologie des Concentrations Minérales Stratiformes*." I tried my best to understand this exclusively French approach to mineral exploration, but it was very academic and outside the understanding of more conventional approaches.

Twelve weeks of continuous field work is too long. Efficiency declines at around the six-week mark. The field work commenced within thick scrub and trees, which was too thick for four-wheel drive penetration. We found that out the hard way. We commenced with two

Landrovers and completely destroyed the lead Landrover in a week. The decision was made to hire a D7 bulldozer and push an access road sixty-kilometres through the heart of the permit. I then had the task of sampling and mapping both sides of the road on foot.

The exploration was performed in part on the Mainoru pastoral lease and an Aboriginal reserve. I had a cook, a mechanic, and a field hand as support. We were required to have an Aboriginal guide as custodian of Aboriginal cultural matters. Jedda was only a sixteen-year-old boy and not well steeped in his Aboriginal knowledge. He came down with chicken pox within the first three weeks of being with us, and the mechanic drove him into his home in Bulman. He was never replaced.

I discovered some remarkable Aboriginal cave paintings, and this happened while Jedda was with me. He showed little interest in them, although to be fair, by this stage he had a temperature as he was coming down with his chicken pox. Those paintings remain the best Aboriginal art I have ever seen; skeletal fish paintings with their internal organs faithfully reproduced. I reported these to the National Museum.

A bushfire had broken out on Mainoru Station that the homestead owner claimed we instigated from a spark caused by our bulldozer's tracks on a rock or by hot cinders from the exhaust pipe. I thought his claim fanciful, but for good relations we suspended our activities to assist him and his stockmen with the fire. It was not a serious fire and we managed to encircle it and starve the life out of it with hessian bags. There was ample light provided by the fire and we worked into the night. When the fire was extinguished the only light remaining was that provided by the stars. I found that I was without a compass and with no knowledge of navigation by the stars, which way to return to our vehicles? Debates broke out between rival and very diverse theories. We were led home by the knowledge of the station owner that the 'panhandle sets in the west.' I stuck with him. The alternate group spent the night in the bush. Because of this incident we had a great relationship with the station owner. From that point on he assisted us in whatever way he could. The access road we left him would have been invaluable for mustering his wandering cattle.

54

TREES DON'T TALK BACK

The Petrel No 1 blowout had caused a pause in Aquitaine's program. Not having an Honours degree, I enrolled in a part time M.Sc. Qualifying degree at the University of Queensland which would allow me to then advance to a Master of Science degree. Study was to be through the completion of the coursework and a thesis. I also managed a football comeback with Western Districts. Team sports did not sit well with the long absences associated with geological fieldwork and my football and cricket had been abandoned.

I started remarkably well with Wests, running backwards and fearlessly taking marks resulting in a couple of best on-the-ground performances and ultimate promotion to the firsts. I had one game at full forward in which I didn't get a kick, so I was immediately dropped back to the seconds. A few games in, it occurred to me that if I keep this up I might get hurt, and so I started to look around and take care of myself. I subsequently lost all form and didn't get much of the ball. This turned out to be a problem for the coach. He knew I could play, but where? He commenced an experimental program with me. I had always either played as a wingman, small forward, or rover. He creatively used me as a back-man, starting me in the back pocket.

We were playing at the Gabba against Morningside. Our fullback was on a big bruiser with bulging tattooed biceps and a pinhead. He took a great mark, and the bruiser came through and clipped him behind the ear quite late. I confronted the bruiser and, with chest out, told him what I thought of his cowardly act. My words must have enraged him. As if in a slow-motion replay, I watched as the bruiser clenched his fist and he gave me one to the face. I dropped to the ground in a daze. The next thing I knew I was looking at my captain's face. He had my shoulders pinned to the ground as he said, 'Don't hit him back, you've got a free kick.' I pretended outrage as I got up and wanted to have the bruiser on but decided to take the free kick, a good sign that my brain was still working.

The coach was exhilarated at my great show of courage, and in the following week I was promoted to centre half back. I had heard all my life that a back-man keeps the ball in front of him and runs through the pack. Great advice, but the trouble was I came out the other side of the pack with a broken collar bone. I ran around with a useless arm for a little while until I looked over at the coach who was shaking his head and remonstrating to me to come off. I was escorted to the waiting ambulance that was parked near the goals. Kathy, now pregnant with our second child, and Nicole were at the game, and as luck had it were alongside the ambulance. The ambo comforted Nicole as I disappeared inside, 'Daddy will be alright, we'll take good care of him.'

I emerged from the hospital with my left arm in a sling for the collar bone break and, as they had discovered I had also broken the little finger in my right hand, I had plaster up to my elbow on that arm. I was useless and would be so for four weeks. Aquitaine was not impressed. Kathy had to attend to all my needs, including going to the toilet. It was not a good situation by any means.

To top it all off, during my convalescence Kathy had to be rushed to give birth just before my arm was due to come out of the sling, and the plaster was to be removed from my other arm. I offered to take my arm out of the sling as I hopped around trying to get my pants on one handed. She took one look at me, and I could see that same disappointed look in her eyes that I had seen in my football coach. She rolled her eyes and shook her head from side to side as she calmly rang one of our neighbours. All I could do was sit in the back seat with her as she held my plastered arm. There was a similar dismissive drop off at the hospital that I had experienced with Nicole's arrival as the Mater nuns took Kathy into her care.

And so, our second daughter Suzie was born. We were now a family of four. When I returned to Aquitaine for work, I received a serious reprimand from the Exploration Manager. "You are a professional. You are expected to be available twenty-four hours a day, seven days a week."

It was the wakeup call I needed for it struck home to me that as the sole breadwinner I needed to be fit and capable. I could not afford to be taking these sorts of risks and be unemployed. His speech had a big influence on my future behaviour. There was to be no football comeback for me, my family was my priority.

****

One of the units I was studying was marine science, and I noticed an opportunity to apply for a Shell Scholarship that ran for two years resulting in an M.Sc. to study at the University of Aberystwyth, majoring in Marine Science.

One night after work, I enthusiastically approached Kathy and asked, 'How would you like two years in Aberystwyth?'

'Where the hell is Aberystwyth?' she asked as she attempted to feed Suzie who was squirming in her high chair.

'It's in Wales.'

'Go on, tell me more,' she replied.

'Well, Shell is offering a scholarship to study for an M.Sc. It takes two years. The money's not great, but we should be able to get by. We would be together every night, and at the end of our time there is the likelihood of a career with Shell.'

Kathy didn't hesitate, 'Okay, have a go at it. Anything is better than this existence.'

I promptly mailed an application. When not in the field and at the head office, I habitually rang Kathy at lunchtime. Two weeks later when I rang home for the lunchtime chat, Nicole answered the phone.

'Hello, gorgeous! Is Mum there?'

'Hi Dad, Mum says she's busy and can't come to the phone,' replied the ever-responsible Nicole.

'Okay Nicki, tell Mum that I'll ring back after I have eaten my sandwiches. Love ya.'

So, when the phone rang a second time, Kathy rushed to the phone and seductively said, 'Hello there big boy. What can I do for you?'

There was a moment of complete silence and then a cultured voice; 'Hello, I am James Polkinghorne from Shell Development Australia. May I speak to Dennis?'

This exchange wasn't the best of starts for my aspirations of winning the scholarship. Kathy had acted outside her character norm. We understood academic ability was not the only attribute Shell was assessing; the successful applicant was to be an ambassador for both Shell and Australia.

Despite this set back, I was selected for an interview which was to be held in a fortnight's time. This was an extraordinarily busy time in my life. I was working full time, studying for the Qualifying degree, working around the house, and maintaining some semblance of a social life. This was compounded in this fortnight with long nights studying for four examination papers for the degree. I normally would keep up with current affairs, but this hectic routine did not allow much time for reading the newspapers.

Accordingly, I was not exactly fresh and alert when I arrived for my interview. Shell had hired a large room at the Hilton Hotel. Three representatives had flown up from Melbourne: James Polkinghorne, Albert, and Michelle. When introduced, I had just enough time to take in that Michelle was very attractive. She had swarthy skin, permed, bouncy jet-black hair with a pert figure and long eyelashes. For a moment, I thought I may have met this girl before?

The room contained one long table with only four chairs. James and Albert were grouped on one side of the table with Michelle positioned right down at the other end.

James was the principal interviewer and took control. 'Take a seat, Dennis.'

I had no choice, the Shell team had prearranged the seating. It was a muggy day in Brisbane, and nervous beads of sweat broke out on my forehead. My peripheral vision was insufficient to see Michelle down the other end of the table. However, I could sense the fluttering of her long eye lashes and could smell her striking perfume.

'Now Dennis, I feel like I already know your wife, having spoken to her on the phone,' James begun.

'Mm,' I muttered.

'Yes, an interesting conversation. So, tell us why you want to study marine geology.'

I had prepared for the series of technical questions very well. I was keen and focussed on my technical goals and growth objectives. I began to relax and was very pleased on how the interview was proceeding. I was on a roll and beginning to think that I was a real chance at winning the scholarship. The technical questions went on for some thirty minutes and then there was a dramatic pause, and my euphoria was broken by Michelle's soft voice from the far end of the table.

'Now Dennis, we would like to take a different tack now.'

I slowly screwed my head to the left to see Michelle and then, remembering my father's wise counsel, "always look people in the eye son," I readjusted my chair to more easily engage with her.

She commenced, 'Do you go to the ABC concerts?'

'The ABC concerts?' I was thinking, *What the hell sort of question is that*?

'Yes,' she replied.

'Err, No,'

'What then is your taste in music?'

I rushed in, 'Oh, I have a very broad taste in music. I love traditional jazz, Dixieland, modern jazz, progressive jazz, funk, and bebop jazz.'

'Mm', she said. This was a knowing sort of demeaning "Mm" and implied this was not quite the answer that she wanted to hear. She lowered her eyes to confer to her papers and then after raising her head, fluttering her eyelashes, and extending her full lips into a sweet smile she asked; 'What do you think about the situation in the Middle East?'

'Oh, the Middle East situation?' Moments passed, it seemed like an eternity. Nothing could assemble in my dull, exhausted, overworked brain.

'W... we... well... I think the Jews are entitled to their little bit of land.'

'Mm, thank you.' I wasn't at all comfortable and sweat sprang up in pores all over my face.

She continued, 'Can you tell me who is the recently appointed Chairman of the Wool Board?'

'The Wood Board?' I queried.

'No Dennis, the Wool Board,' she slowly enunciated as though I was a simpleton. Her lips weren't smiling now.

'Oh, the Wool Board,' I responded as though this clarified the question. I was trying in desperation to stall for time. 'The Wool Board, Ah... um... No.' I bumbled out.

'Thank you, Dennis. No more questions from me, James,' Michelle said as she energetically ticked off notes on her writing pad.

James finalised the interview, 'Well, Dennis, thank you for coming in. We will let you know if you have been selected. Don't bother to ring us, we'll ring you.'

Totally deflated, I mumbled some sort of thank you and closing statement before leaving the room. I couldn't wait to get away and back into the field. At least the trees don't talk to you like these Shell gorillas. Dejectedly, I left the Hilton and walked to the next closest hotel bar. As I perched on a stool I laid each of the Shell business cards on the bar. One read 'Michelle Frydenberg - Corporate Lawyer.'

Slowly, I remembered where I had met Michelle before. She was my Elwood High School rival. I looked into my glass and asked no one in particular, 'How the hell will I make prime minister?'

The barman responded, 'Who in their right mind wants to be prime minister?'

'Can I have another beer? A large one?' I asked.

55

YOURS TRULY SHUTS DOWN NT RAILWAYS

I was not smart enough to know that I was on a good wicket with Aquitaine, an international oil company. Desperate for a few extra dollars for my expanding family, in 1971 I joined Thiess as a coal exploration geologist. Thiess was an earth moving company and showed little respect for professional geologists. Being poorly treated and not finding coal a stimulating commodity, I looked around for alternative employment. I was only nine months with Thiess before I resigned and joined the Frances Creek Iron Mining Corporation (FIMCO), a privately-owned company running an iron ore mine in the Northern Territory.

'At least I'll be home every night,' I told Kathy. 'Go bush young man and make your fortune was the plan.' So, we sold our first home and banked the money. The only problem with this plan was that it coincided with Gough Whitlam's loss of control of the Australian economy. Annual inflation ran at over fifteen percent in both 1974 and 1975. Apart from the short post war spike, this was the greatest inflation spike ever experienced in Australia. We would have done better financially to be on the dole and watch the value of our house inflate. I could have started my other career, becoming a writer, but would I have accrued the same life experiences? 'A resounding no,' is the answer to that question. I was not to know at the time, but I was to precipitate the closure of the complete Northern Territory railways for three days.

****

'Alex, I am sorry, but you leave me no alternative, you're sacked. I have given you three prior warnings which you have ignored, and on this last occasion you've put a life at risk,' I pronounced.

Alex looked aghast, in total shock. He picked himself up and left the room. How had it come to this? Alexander Popov was Polish but thankfully not of the same stature as Alf, my former Polish school friend.

FIMCO was a non-listed company developing the small iron ore deposits at Frances Creek. Frances Creek is about twenty-six kilometres north east of Pine Creek and approximately one hundred and eighty-five kilometres south east of Darwin. To the south some one hundred and seventeen kilometres on the Stuart Highway was the centre of Katherine. Even by the standards of existing iron ore mines back in the 70's this was a very small iron ore operation, targeting one million tonnes of produced ore per annum. For a variety of reasons, the mine never reached that target. The ore was a high-grade hematite with some specular varieties providing great "specimen" quality pieces for collectors.

While Gough Whitlam was fighting off Malcolm Fraser in Canberra, I had my own battles to fight in Frances Creek. In 1972 there were two geologists on site, one being a Canadian mining geologist to whom I reported. Not unrelated to decisions of the Whitlam government and a souring economy, I was approached by the FIMCO Managing Director with the words,

'We don't mind if you look for another job, Dennis. Things are very tight with the company right now.'

I had to think fast, there were mouths to feed. This was not a good time to be out of a job. Some of my geologist friends were driving taxis and assembling Brownbuilt cabinets.

'Listen, if you want this job done I am your man. I know how to work and get things done,' I claimed.

Within a fortnight my boss was driving out of town with his family.

There was no qualified mining engineer on site, so I was thrown a text book on open cut mine planning and given the task of designing extraction mining plans for the multi-pit operation. It was an exacting task that just had to be completed on time. I was now Chief Geologist. More accurately, I was the only geologist. My department consisted of a draftsman, a surveyor, and two surveyor assistants. Most workers passing through Frances Creek were transients from "down south," either running away from the law or women. Surveyor assistants were typical of these workers. Many were on drugs. At various times, the department had "Clip-On Eye Balls," thankfully he only had to hold the surveyor's staff not look through the theodolite, "No Worries", permanently recovering from inebriation, "Hazy" and "Alex", to name but a few.

Friday night was film night at the Recreation Centre, or the "Club" as it was called. Films were projected onto a pull-down screen in the open air. One night, while viewing a particularly tense film in which a bully was terrorising people in a train carriage, "No Worries" could take no more of the building tension, and he punched the villain on the screen. There was a big hole in the screen, the lights went on, the camera wound down, and "No Worries" was restrained.

"Hazy," a drug challenged individual with strange but permanent horizons across his eyes, could normally be found seated cross-legged behind the surveyor's office door using yarrow stacks to consult the "I Ching." You could never tell if his eyes were rising or setting over his strange horizons.

Alexander Popov was of greater sobriety than the others, a long-term employee and a friend of the mine manager. He had taken on extra voluntary duties such as emergency first aid officer when Leslie, the mine nurse, was off-site.

Arriving on duty one morning, I had just parked my vehicle when on rounding the corner of the office block, I was accosted by "Hazy".

'I got crabs,' he said.

'Oh, really,' I replied. It was not quite what I wanted to hear straight after my Weetbix and before my day's work. 'Why not go to Leslie or Alex.'

'Well, they're both off-site today and you're the next first aid officer.' "Hazy" was correct in this. I was the second on-site first aid officer, backing up Leslie and Alex. So quirkily Alex, who reported to me as part of my department, had seniority in first aid support.

'Okay, come with me and I'll ring the nurse at Pine Creek to see what we should do,' I responded.

"R&R" had become a common term throughout the Vietnam War in which Australia was involved from 1966 to 1972. I was part of the birthday ballot but luckily my birth date was not drawn out. The term was adopted at the mine site. Staff and key personnel were allowed "rest and recreation" leave once a month to go to Darwin for some essential shopping, stock up on supplies, and have a break from the mine site.

At the peak of its productive life, Frances Creek had a workforce of one hundred and a population of two hundred, counting children. The town consisted of twenty-five houses, barrack accommodation for single men, and a caravan park. As well as the "Club" there was a small general store at which the workers could buy food on credit, chalked up against their next pay packet. We had a staff house and it just so happened that our next-door neighbours were Alex and his partner.

I called Alex to my office, 'Alex, I don't mind you going on R&R but I need to know that you are taking it and that you are not on site. You know this is the third time we have had this discussion. Just show me the courtesy of telling me, will you?'

'Sure, Dennis,' Alex sheepishly replied. 'It won't happen again.'

It did happen again and only one month after the Hazy 'crabs' incident. There was general panic at the mine site office.

Bleeker Groote, the Administration Manager, burst into my office. 'Dennis, Biggsie's son Bert has swallowed some turps. Leslie's on R&R, and we cannot find Alex. You're next man on duty,' he panted.

'Shit. Alex hasn't left me with the ambulance keys.'

Bleeker Groote ran off to locate the reserve set of ambulance keys. I rang the Katherine Base Hospital to get instructions.

The nurse advised, 'Get him to drink several glasses of water. Do not let him throw up. Get the young fellow here as quick as possible and keep him warm and quiet.'

'It's going to take about an hour and a half to get there,' I said.

'Best to not delay,' she responded.

As I hung up, Bleeker Groote rushed back jangling the keys, 'Found them, you better scoot.'

'Yep, I'll let you know when I have delivered him to the hospital.'

I collected young Bert Biggs. At four years old he was anything but big. His mother and I strapped him to the stretcher and we took off. She rode in the back with Bert. Heart pumping, adrenalin flowing, a life-threatening emergency sharpens every fibre in the body. There can be no failure here. I reprimanded myself to stay alert and concentrate. I was thinking all sorts of what ifs, what if this, what if that. My first aid training had been quite basic.

Fortunately, the trip passed without incident. Bert's mother had done a wonderful job keeping her son quiet, and he had kept down two large glasses of water. They both stayed in the hospital, and I returned to Frances Creek alone and exhausted. My mind was still active however as on the return trip I started to think where the hell had Alex been? It should have been Alex on duty, in charge of this incident. The more I mulled it over the angrier I became. If he hasn't got a valid explanation, well...

That evening, the welcome news was received at the mine that young Bert was stable and out of danger. There was great relief and the downing of celebratory drinks to young Bert's health at the 'Club'. Alex was nowhere to be seen.

The next morning Alex appeared, jittery and shifty-eyed.

'What's the story, Alex?'

'Ah, ah I went up to Darwin for some R&R.'

'You didn't tell me. You've had three prior warnings.'

'Yes, I'm sorry.'

'Well, I am sorry too, but you leave me no alternative, you're sacked. I have given you three prior warnings which you have ignored, and on this last occasion you've put a life at risk. Young Bert Biggs could have died you know.'

'You're not for real, are you?'

'This has been a very serious incident. It's all over for you. Go and see Bleeker Groote, and he'll work out your termination payout.'

Alex looked aghast, in total shock. He picked himself up and left the room. How had it come to this? He had developed a personal friendship at the top with the mine manager. Unfortunately for Alex, the mine manager was on extended annual leave for six weeks. A young mining engineer had been brought in under contract to fill in for the mine manager.

Alex wasn't going to take this on the chin. He refused to admit any wrong doing. Appeal to the Union was the next step. This took a day to organise.

Once mobilised, and only hearing Alex's side of the dismissal, the workers went out on strike. Initially, the workers were represented by the local NT Union representative, Paddy Carroll.

Now, I was of the habit of driving home from the mine site office to have lunch with the family. It meant of course driving past Alex and his partner's house. As I drove home for lunch on the second day, a large gathering of workers had collected under the house the other side of Alex's. My God, what is this? I thought. God, it's a Union meeting. Don't look left, you might get skinned alive or pelted with eggs.

Alexander Popov, because of his longevity at the mine, had worked at some time or other in each of the other departments. It had been suggested by Paddy Carroll that Alex be reinstated in another department other than Geology and Surveying. Each of the department heads, when asked, resisted. They did not want to have anything more to do with him. In one way or another they had all been burnt by this guy in the past. There was a healthy stock pile of mined and crushed iron ore that could be loaded on the daily iron ore train to Darwin for export at the port terminal. The staff was quite capable of loading the trains and were in fact enjoying being 'boys' again with all the hands-on work. It was an escape from their normal supervisory work.

This was not going well for the workers, and it was starting to affect their families in the town as credit was withdrawn from the 'General Store.' Not only did I have to endure the intense worker stares from meetings under the Union house, but Kathy was now feeling most uncomfortable as she purchased produce from the General Store.

It was now day nine, and the negotiations were at an impasse and it seemed to be beyond Paddy Carroll. The local union decided to fly an AWU heavy weight from Melbourne to take over negotiations. He had presided over significant industrial disputes. He was also physically heavy. Now I found myself alongside the acting manager, who was only some five years older than me, on one side of the table faced off against Paddy Carroll and the heavy weight. The only industrial relations experience we had was negotiating with our respective wives with limited success at that. This was a mismatch from the outset. Why hadn't FIMCO flown up some of their Sydney management team for these negotiations? I was wishing that Michelle Frydenberg was sitting alongside me right now.

There was little listening going on in this negotiation, the heavy weight was determined to drive the whole conversation. Slouched in his chair with cigarette in hand, he shifted his ample frame and trumpeted, 'This is the way it is, you cannot summarily dismiss such a long-term employee of the mine.'

'You do understand that his actions threatened a child's life, do you not?' stated my manager.

'You're being melodramatic,' countered the Unionist.

'Well, you weren't driving the bloody ambulance for ninety minutes. It was touch and go,' I contributed, anger rising.

The discussion escalated quickly, 'Listen and listen carefully, this thing could go national,' the heavy weight said as he leaned forward to eyeball us. He continued, 'Before we go national, I'm going to shut down the Northern Territory railways. You've seen the last of your trains getting out of Frances Creek until you reinstate Popov.' At that he rose from his chair saying, 'Come on Paddy, nothing more to do here,' and he rocked from the room.

I slammed the front door of the house as I returned home and said, 'The bloody standover bastards are threatening to shut down the NT railways, not just the Frances Creek spur line but the whole bloody NT railways. Do you believe it?'

Kathy did her best to calm me down. 'Don't worry, better that he's standing over you than sitting on you.'

'Oh, very funny. This is no time for humour.'

'Quieten down, will you? You'll wake the children. Come and have a drink, it'll be better in the morning.'

The threat became fact the next day. All traffic on the NT rail network ceased. Bleeker Groote gathered the department heads together.

'Guys, it looks like we might just have to re-employ Alex. Who's prepared to have him?' Bleeker asked.

Each one stated, some with very colourful language, that they wouldn't have Alex in their department.

'Okay. I guess we sweat it out then,' Bleeker said. 'We'll get together again tomorrow morning at nine o'clock.'

The stalemate continued for another two days. A strange quiet descended on the remote mining town. Credit had also been cut off at the "Club". This was an incendiary powder keg waiting to erupt – men, NT men, cut off from their grog. The ever present red dust had settled on the roads as no cars moved nor did the mining equipment operate.

On the third morning, Bleeker called the department heads together again.

'This is how it is. I have had instructions from the directors. This is just too costly, they cannot hold out any longer. I have to place Alex back in the workforce,' Bleeker stated.

'Fine, but who is going to take him?' asked one of the Department heads.

'As none of you want him and I have my instructions from the directors, he's coming on as an administration assistant under me,' he replied. 'Now that you have been informed, I am going down to the town to inform Paddy Carroll.'

I ran out to my car and quickly drove into the town behind Bleeker.

Bursting into the house, I spat out the words to Kathy, 'The company has caved in, they are putting Alex back on staff as an administration assistant under Bleeker. I feel sick, let's get out of town and have some R&R in Darwin.'

'No, no man of mine is going to leave town with his tail between his legs. You just go about your work as though nothing has changed. You have more supporters in this town than you know,' Kathy replied.

I stepped down quickly, 'You're right, thanks love.' This was just another negotiation I had lost. I was a good geologist but an unlikely prime minister.

56

CAREER MOVES

The Frances Creek Mine ran into some problems. Benches on my mine plans were being mined out quicker than they should have been. The ore had been defined on percussion drilling only, and the sample interval had been such that the ore had been overstated. FIMCO management assigned Thiess Constructions to take over the management of the mine.

Thiess contracted some consulting geologists who I assisted to undertake a diamond core drill program which established the correct reserves of the mine. The result was a dramatic reduction in reserves. The writing was on the wall for the mine, and I immediately commenced looking for another job. As a preference I targeted positions in Melbourne. I made the interview for two, and I managed to organise the interviews on successive days. One was with Shell for a position as a Coal Geologist, and the other was with Jennings Mining Ltd, a subsidiary of AV Jennings, the successful home building company. I was, thankfully (because the thought of coal was not exciting), rejected by Shell. Probably Michelle Frydenberg had informed Human Resources that I was a big risk.

I accepted the position of Research Geologist with Jennings. They wanted me for my sedimentary skills. Kathy and I had managed to escape from Frances Creek, with paid airfares and removal costs.

I did some of my best field mapping projects while with Jennings, as Project Leader looking for lead-zinc in carbonates in the Buchan Basin, and copper-uranium in red beds of the Mansfield Basin. Both basins are in Victoria. Another detailed mapping project that I enjoyed was at Errinundra in East Gippsland. This was an 'Irish base metals' limestone-volcanics project. In the height of the summer months, I was conducting traverses over steep, heavily timbered, mountainous terrain. I was wearing heavy denim jeans to help protect my legs from tree and scrub scratches as well as any aggression from the 'limestone' brown snakes. My field season ended painfully with a swollen, red, and infected scrotum. The constant sweating, abrasion of striding uphill, together with the resistant, non-aerated, denim jeans had caused the problem. I had to adopt a bandy-legged walk like a rodeo rider who had just dismounted from a bucking bull. I was dismissed by the doctor with some antibacterial cream. To this day, I detest jeans and the non-breathing nature of denim. Give me cotton duck weave any day.

Jennings Mining was a highly successful group. It had discovered the heavy mineral beach sand deposits of Eneabba and the Argyle diamonds. AV Jennings, however, decided to remain with their core business of building and they shut down their mineral division. The Argyle diamond project was sold off for twenty million dollars. I was retrenched.

My next position was as Resident Geologist for Occidental Minerals of Australia in Perth. I worked from a home office reporting to an Exploration Manager in Sydney. I was duped into thinking this was a senior role. On interview, I was assured that I could employ subcontractors to conduct some of the hard field work, but when it came down to it the Exploration Manager required me to do the lot. I was a one-man band, putting in grid lines, conducting magnetometer traverses, and supervising drilling operations. I was in the field two weeks in three for the full year. It was no life for Kathy and the children. We now had our third daughter, Tess. Tess was born at the Mercy Hospital in Melbourne. Kathy had the heavy load of running the home almost single-handedly because of my long absences. On the weeks when I was home, I was exhausted, recovering from the last field trip, writing it up, and preparing for the next assignment.

Working alone in the bush is quite disconcerting. What if you should have an accident or have a vehicle breakdown? On assignment in Cue, on the Western Australian shield, I would notify the local policeman where I was working for the day, so that if I did not present myself to the police station the following day, they would have some idea of where to come looking for me. There were no mobile phones back then.

I was on assignment in Leonora working from the Leonora Motel. After a day's work it was worth a drink in the Leonora pub just to view the latest gold nugget that the amateur fossickers had discovered with their metal detectors. I had never seen so much gold, and each nugget had its own character which is why they have been given names throughout history. The one I distinctly remember was shaped like an elephant and was the size of my thumb down to the first knuckle.

Over a beer in the pub I could reflect on where I was at with this career of mine. I had started in soft rock as a petroleum geologist and had migrated from coal, to sedimentary iron ore, and into a hard rock base metals explorationist. Trouble was that all the green, metamorphosed, deeply weathered, rocks of the Western Australian shield all looked the same to me, and I was meant to be able to distinguish between them. I had reached the same wall I felt when studying Pure Mathematics II all those years ago. I felt bewildered, swamped, overcome, and lost all in one.

Kathy knew the near desperate state I was in, and I needed an out. We both had endured two years of hard labour. It was she who noticed the advertisement in the paper. Beach Petroleum had a position for a Junior Petroleum Geologist based in Melbourne. I applied for the position from the Leonora Motel.

I won the position, but there were two problems. One was that at the age of thirty-one starting in a junior role, I had to basically turn around and retrain myself all over again to become an effective petroleum geologist. For the last eight years I had been a mineral geologist. The harder problem was that of my parents.

When Dad and Mum came home from Greece, they landed in Darwin and visited us at the Frances Creek iron ore mine. Dad looked dreadful, grey and drawn and fighting for breath all the time. He still managed his 'I'm alright, Jack, nothing wrong here' persona, but families know, don't they? Family knows the best and the worst of its members.

They returned to the family home in Glen Iris and shortly afterwards Kathy, the children, and I returned to Melbourne when I won the Jennings job. Three years later when we went to Perth for the job with Occidental, Mum and Dad sold the Melbourne home and moved to Perth as well. It was their home state and they had Aunt Joy, some of Mum's sisters and brother, and friends there, but I felt that our move had been the catalyst. I was filled with grief and guilt when I had to announce to them that the Occidental job had been pure hell for me and that we were upping stakes again and off to Melbourne. Dad took it on the chin like all things. 'Dennis, you've got your own life to sort out. Toss you up in the air and you always land on your feet. You'll be prime minister one day, son,' he said in between wheezes.

I went home and wept for him, and wept for us. 'Why does life have to be so hard?' I felt like I had deserted him, let him down. This man had carried the burden of the family on his shoulders for so long and he was now a depleted, sick entity still resolutely shouldering on, walking the tightrope to protect his wife from too much stress and social exposure. I should have been there supporting him, giving him and Mum exposure to their grandchildren, adding value to their lives. However, I thought I had no alternative but to chase work to feed our blossoming family which now numbered five. Up until now, I had five different jobs over eleven years and Kathy and I had lived in four different states. That's not a particularly great average.

57

THE CARAVAN STORY

One of my lucky breaks in life was re-joining the soft rock Petroleum fraternity, even if I was starting at the bottom rung all over again. Being married with children and with some maturity I could focus and apply myself completely to the task of learning the complexities of my chosen profession.

Beach Petroleum was a unique, small Australian explorer with a technical team of four: Exploration Manager, Petroleum Engineer, Geophysicist, and myself as the new Geologist recruit with support administrative staff. The company had been founded by Dr Reg Sprigg, a highly decorated, respected, and exceptional geologist. I regard him as the father of the Australian oil patch, and he was the foundation president of APEA, the Australian Petroleum Exploration Association. APEA ran annual conferences where technical advances and discoveries were shared. It was also a lobby group to government, advancing geologic knowledge to the nation.

I was fortunate to have an office alongside Reg, and I was exposed to his technical brilliance, bright creative mind, and motivated by his enthusiasm for the search for oil. Beach was unique at the time as it fully owned and operated all its acreage. From my point of view, this was outstanding, and I embarked on a steep learning curve.

Beach held the whole onshore Otway Basin under exploration license. Our Exploration Manager, Ian MacPhee, knew the basin well from his time employed as a geologist with the Victorian Mines Department. He had developed 'plays,' concepts of where oil might be located, and within what rock formations. I was trained up as a well site geologist for the upcoming drilling program by a very experienced mud logger. There is no better way to learn to become a petroleum geologist than to 'sit' on wells as they are drilled. It brings the whole science alive to the essential elements of the game.

Ian MacPhee had a press clipping framed in his office, the headline of which was, 'Otway Basin is Dry: Shell.' Shell, the major international company, after considerable review and expenditure had written the Otway Basin off as not likely to be petroliferous, and had abandoned their search. Ian thought differently and was determined to prove them wrong.

Up until the North Paaratte-1 well, which spudded near Port Campbell in October 1979, Beach had participated in sixty unsuccessful wells over eighteen years in the Australian oil patch. I was the well site geologist for Beach and called the drill stem test that flowed seven million cubic feet per day. The flare was lit by throwing a burning rag in front of the flow line and there was a thunderous, deafening roar. This was to be Beach's first commercial discovery after all those years of endeavour, and I had the good fortune to be involved with the discovery. The field and subsequent adjacent discoveries were developed to supply Warrnambool with enough gas for over twenty years. It was both a technical and a commercial triumph.

I obtained a copy of Ian's press clipping of Shell's misguided pronouncement on the potential of the basin and placed it in a frame on my desk. For motivation each morning I would raise it up, look it in the eye, and proclaim, 'Here's looking at you, Michelle.'

****

'Hey, Dennis. Triton's in town, do you feel like lunch?' asked Ian, the Beach Exploration Manager.

'Sure Ian,' I replied feeling quite elevated, 'love to.'

'Only thing is, you have to tell the caravan story,' he chuckled.

'Sure thing, my pleasure,' I gracefully replied. I could always be bought by a good meal.

These were the heady days of the world oil price bubble of the late 1970s, early 1980s. Even senior geologists can dine out on shareholder funds in booms, and junior oil companies like Beach could enjoy head offices in Collins Street, Melbourne. But I well knew that there were no free lunches and this one would be well earned in telling the caravan story.

By August 1980 my career was progressing well. Now in my twelfth year, I had served my apprenticeship and had the lofty title of Senior Geologist in charge of Beach's Surat exploration program. I could share my knowledge with the next generation of geologists. I was training Robin, the latest fledgling straight out of University entrusted to my care, in the craft of being a well site geologist. Beach's latest Surat Basin exploration well, Toorumbee-1, was forty-three kilometres east of St George and two kilometres south of the Moonie Highway, on the floodplain of the Moonie River.

As we strode around the well site, we were referred to, in the good bush Aussie, humorous way, as Batman and Robin. 'You have to learn to roll with this Robin. I was once run off a well site by a drunk drilling engineer. When I appealed to Ian, he just said to go back tomorrow morning, he won't have any memory of it.'

In the normal chain of command on a well site, the drilling engineer is in charge of drilling the well to its' total depth (TD) and the geologist is responsible for all other important decisions of where to call tests, where to cut cores, stop drilling to circulate bottoms up, and calling TD.

'We are here to evaluate, the engineer is here to get to TD as quick and as cheaply as possible, so there is always conflict,' I advised, feeling very much like the old hand. On this well I had the added responsibility of being the most senior Beach representative as the drilling engineer was a consultant.

Drilling is a twenty-four hour activity. It doesn't stop just because the geologist might be tired. Working hours are irregular; no unionism here, no standard days. It takes whatever it takes to keep up and you must be up to date for the morning report to head office. No excuses. No problem for the drilling crew, they work in two separate twelve-hour shifts.

'Robin, this game is all about prediction based on theory followed by observation and then revision of your theories, repeated over and over again. Flexibility, Robin, flexibility. Got to always be able to touch your toes,' I said, acting the eccentric as I touched my toes.

As the drill bit turns, the latest piece of information is transferred to the surface as drill cuttings by the mud system and are examined by the geologist.

Drilling success in this part of the Surat Basin was only about five percent. That is ninety-five percent of wells have no oil and are declared dry. They are not completed but are plugged and abandoned. In these wells, cement plugs are set in the well bore to avoid the mixing of different formation waters. And so it passed with Toorumbee-1. After twelve days of drilling and the calling of one drill stem test there was not a whiff of hydrocarbons, so now for abandonment. But before abandonment, the geologist must manage the maximisation of data collection on the well and ensure that the running of the electric logs, run by a third-party service company, is done properly and that they are of suitable quality. Beach had elected to trial a smaller, new contractor on Toorumbee-1. I had argued against this at the planning stage but had lost the argument.

The decision resulted in a nightmare. Every tool the contractor ran in the well failed. It just produced meaningless electrical squiggles. It was impossible for me to get any sleep at all. Each tool took three to four hours of running in and out of the hole and I was required to examine and ultimately approve the acceptability and quality of the results. The logging exercise took two days instead of the usual nine hours. I had no sleep throughout and was forced to compromise on one important log by substituting a less desirable one.

'Now listen, Robin. This is the plan. As the company rep, I need to observe that the cement plugs have been placed correctly and are set. I'm pulling rank mate, you can drive the Toyota and the caravan back to Melbourne, but I'm flying home. I have worked out that there is a flight out of Moree at seven o'clock tomorrow morning. The plugs should be set at about midnight, so if we drive through the night I'll be able to make it. It's only a two- hundred and fifty-kilometre drive. You go and hook the caravan up, ready for a quick getaway. I have to be up on the drill floor with the drilling engineer.'

'Sure, Batman,' Robin said. Even he was starting to lose the plot.

As had been repeatedly affirmed on Toorumbee-1, everything took longer than anticipated, so it wasn't until two in the morning that we could pull out.

'I'll drive, and then you'll be fresh to drive on from Moree,' I said. Tentatively we picked our way along the initial forty-kilometres of narrow dirt track. It was mostly a straight track except I do recall slowing down on a curve before a cattle grid, doing little more than a crawl, followed by a gentle descent to cross the Moonie River. Shortly after the creek crossing, I came to a stop and said, 'Time for a pit stop.'

We both walked away from the Toyota and relieved ourselves, and then walked back and hopped into the vehicle. After that, we took a right turn onto the Barwon Highway bitumen. There was not much banter between us as we were both dog tired. After a further fifteen kilometres we took a left-hand turn onto the Carnarvon Highway. I was driving very carefully due to my fatigue and took the turn very slowly. As I began to settle into the easier bitumen driving I turned to Robin and said, 'You know these Toyota's are fabulous, aren't they? They are so powerful you wouldn't even know if you're towing a caravan.' No sooner were the words out of my mouth when I glanced at the rear vision mirror, 'Bloody hell! Where's the caravan?' Incredulously, I braked sharply and got out of the vehicle just to confirm that there was no caravan.

'What are we going to do? You put the safety chains on, didn't you?' I asked.

'Yes, of course I did,' Robin responded.

'Well, we've just got to go find it,' I muttered through clenched teeth. I turned the Toyota around and started the search by slowly retracing our steps. I was having visions of the caravan just flying off onto the flat Moonie River floodplain. It could go for miles before it might come to a stop. Alternatively, it could just be in a crumpled hump somewhere. Even worse, how do you report to head office that you've lost a caravan? I could imagine just how well that conversation would go.

We crawled north peering into the early dawn light looking for the caravan. It was after I had repeated for the umpteenth time,

'What are we going to tell the head office?' that Robin cracked back, 'How wouldn't you know you weren't towing the caravan?'

We had been a good team up until then. I bit my lip and responded, 'Let's not go there, Robin. I know I had the van when I turned onto the bitumen.' Shortly after that remark we arrived at the junction of the bitumen and the dirt track. There was nothing for it but to drive back up the dirt track.

Still edging along and peering into the bush, we both recognised where we had stopped and relieved ourselves. 'Surely, we had the van at that point,' I commented. Robin was mute.

Then we crossed the Moonie River and in the centre of the road on the cattle grid crossing where we had slowed to a crawl sat the caravan. Not a scratch on it. It was obvious what had happened. Robin had forgotten to attach the safety chains to the tow bar, and the ball catch had popped open as the tow bar bottomed on the elevated grid.

We were so elated that we didn't waste energy on recriminations. We both had wounds to lick.

'Listen Robin, not a word to head office about this stuff up, okay?'

'Agreed,' he responded.

Obviously, I didn't catch the plane flight home. Our secret only lasted until the following Christmas party when I decided to tell our story. By sharing the story, I received countless Collins Street lunch invites from Ian. I accepted them all until one morning Ian asked,

'Hey, Dennis. Shell's in town, do you feel like lunch?' Ian asked.

'Who are their reps, Ian?'

'James Polkinghorne and Michelle Frydenberg.'

'Oh, thanks Ian, but I'll take a raincheck on this one. Have to buy something for Kathy's birthday.'

58

UNCLE TED'S LESSONS FINALLY PAY OFF

My career as a geologist cut across my leisure sporting interests. My preferred games of football and cricket are team games, and with long periods of being in the field I could not give valued time to any teams. Aged twenty-four, I had exited football in a spectacular fashion with broken limbs and a warning from the Aquitaine Exploration Manager. From that warning came the realisation that family came first. Now thirty-two years old, I made a cricket comeback. I was invited by Beach's CEO, whom I had befriended, to play with the Heathmont Uniting A grade team who competed in the Ringwood and District League. It was a matting competition which was unusual for me since all of my prior experience had been on turf wickets.

I resumed my role as a sedate opening batsman with the goal to wear the lead bowlers down and protect the flashier batsmen to come. In my first year back in the game I averaged my customary fifteen runs with one fifty. Looking the responsible type in the following year, I was promoted to captain the side and did so for two consecutive seasons. This was an enjoyable time for me and a vindication of all the effort Uncle Ted had put into my cricket development as a youngster.

The game had changed over the twelve years I had been out of it while doing my intensive field work. Grace and good sportsmanship had disappeared and been replaced with mindless sledging promoted at the highest level by the likes of Ian Chappell, Rod Marsh, Dennis Lillee, and co. I deplored this era. Back in 1974 I was in the western stand for the opening day at the MCG Boxing Day test match against England. The Poms lost the series one win to four losses and were terrorised by the fast bowling of Lillee and Jeff Thompson, who bowled with an unusual sling shot action, and on top of that the Australians insulted them with verbal abuse led and endorsed by the captain, Ian Chappell. Due to the number of top line batsmen that had endured injuries from the vicious pummelling received from Lillee and Thompson, the Poms flew out Colin Cowdrey, a forty-one-year old veteran, former champion, and a stylish, graceful, batsman, to help bolster the side. Was this era Australia's comeback against the Poms for their Bodyline assault against Bradman? It sure felt like it.

Colin Cowdrey had lost his youthful physique and there had to be some decline due to age in his reflexes, but years of application to batting technique and its mastery shone through. He came in when England were one down for four runs and faced the venom of Lillee and Thompson bowling at their freshest and fastest. From consecutive bullets slung at him by Thompson, he was hit on the chest and the elbow and fell to the ground. The intoxicated yobbo crowd in the stand above me wildly barracked, pulled tops off beer cans, and with spray descending all over me, mindlessly, obscenely, yelled, 'Knock his bloody head off.' This was in an era before the use of helmets for batsmen. Did any of them understand the enormous courage, concentration, and skill required to face these fast bowlers?

Cowdrey defied the onslaught for two hundred and twenty-nine minutes, faced one hundred and seventy-one balls and scored thirty-five runs. His contribution to the ultimate drawn game was the greatest of any of the players on either side. I have never gone to watch a test match since, preferring to watch it in the comfort of my own home.

With that background in mind, here I was captaining a Uniting Church side called Heathmont which contained players who were mimicking the sledging of Chappell, Marsh, Lillee and co. It surprised me that this church-based club would be into abusive sledging. What, can they just rock up to church the next day and all is forgiven? It is up to the captain to set the tone in which the game is played, both out on the field and in the clubhouse. I pulled my players into line whenever they attempted any sledging. They, at times, were probably surprised but a better game was the result.

In my first year as captain I scored my one and only century. I batted all day and scored one hundred and thirty-two not out. I was concentrating so hard that when I heard some unusual applause from the sidelines I only vaguely registered that maybe I had made a century. I accumulated the second highest number of runs for the team over the season for an average of thirty-two and participated in three of the highest wicket partnerships. I had led the team from the front.

None of my family was there to see my moment of glory, but Uncle Ted would have been so proud. I had lived on potential most of my life and finally I was delivering, well site geologist on a discovery well and a century. Prime ministership could be just around the corner.

I only had one more season after the century with Heathmont. I averaged thirty, participated in two highest wicket partnerships, and had a top score of sixty-eight. Again, the demands of my career took over, and at thirty-five years of age I retired from the game.

59

MORE CAREER MOVES

After three years in the happy and successful camp at Beach Petroleum I was attracted by more money and a title, Chief Petroleum Geologist of Alliance Oil Development, another small Australian oil explorer. At least this did not involve another interstate move, and I had a team of three geologists.

Alliance was such a contrast to Beach as they had a larger spread of acreage with smaller participating interests. This involved more joint venture partners, management, and meetings. Our most important joint venture was with Santos and other companies in the Cooper Basin. The Cooper Basin is Australia's premier onshore oil basin, and the lion's share of the basin was held by Santos and Delhi who shared operatorship between production and exploration. Later, Santos would take over operatorship of both. Alliance held a majority share of fifty percent in the Merrimelia-Innamincka block, one of many blocks across the large PEL 5 & 6 exploration licences. This asset became my principal responsibility, and I commenced attending the monthly Unit Technical Operating Committee (UTOC) meetings in Adelaide. Up to twenty to thirty technical representatives, geologists and engineers from all the joint venture companies would attend these meetings. The operators would present drilling programmes and reserve reviews. As participants we would be alert to decisions that would affect our representative companies. I learnt quickly the skill to argue forcefully for anything that would benefit Alliance and against anything that would be to the detriment of the company. It was similar to politics.

I taught young Robin well site geology, and in return he introduced me to a programmable calculator, a Texas Instrument

59. And so started my fascination with petrophysics, or log analysis. This speciality satisfied my latent love of mathematics. Electrical tools are lowered into the well and upon retrieval record all sorts of rock properties. Petrophysics is the science of interpreting the electrical logs.

From the logs are determined the types of rocks and their reservoir quality, both holding capacity and producibility, and importantly their fluid content, whether that be oil, gas or water. I found this science intriguingly interesting. At the pinnacle of the UTOC debates was the biennial determination of the participation factors of all the joint venture companies in the production revenues from their blocks. This was undertaken in a process referred to as the 'Review and Adjustment'. Petrophysics was an essential component of the Review and Adjustment which would ultimately lead to the distribution of money to each of the participating companies. This work therefore had a direct and immediate impact on company profitability.

Like so much of my work throughout my career, I would tackle problems from first principles. Verification of facts and careful checking of premises is essential, for to do otherwise is to simply perpetuate error or duplicate another person's opinion or position. I advanced both Alliance and my own petrophysical capability by forming a joint venture with the emerging computer company Mincom. Working on my specifications for a log analysis package was the germination of their most successful commercial package, Geolog. During my tenure at Alliance we developed a technical independence that provided an audit to the Operator, ultimately, Santos. Having a controlling interest in the Merrimelia-Innamincka block also aggravated Santos. These factors and the aggression with which I drove the program I believe contributed to Santos' ultimate takeover of Alliance. We were a major thorn in their side and stood in the way of their ambition to control the whole basin.

Santos mounted their takeover of the minor companies within the Cooper Basin Joint Venture. Alliance was the first and messiest of their takeovers. It took over six months to complete. I was forced to work cooperatively with the Santos Exploration Director.

As the termination date approached, the Exploration Director offered me the position of Exploration Manager of Santos Queensland permits, based in their Brisbane office. This would have been a big and prestigious role to undertake, and the offer demanded that I keep my ego in check. Red flags fluttered in my face, I had seen too much of this Exploration Director's ruthless management style. Another opportunity presented itself.

'I'll make sure you won't walk the streets,' Neil said as we sipped our beers. Neil Gantry was Exploration Manager of Crusader Oil, a small Australian oil exploration company based in Brisbane. He was a big, gregarious individual, built like a whale with Valentino hair brushed straight back plastered to his head. He not only had a geology degree but also a legal degree. He was the most outspoken critic of Santos in the UTOC meetings and drove the debates. He understood the politics and the economics of the technical operation so much better than anyone else. I had admired his prowess and standing in the industry, particularly his deal making ability. He was a leader, a mover and a shaker, and he would command attention as he jovially drove technical discussion. Neil attracted, cajoled, and manipulated others to his way of thinking.

'I like the way you stand up for Alliance at UTOC. You understand the geology and petrophysics so well, but more importantly you intuit the best position for your company. Let me work on it. We might be able to create a position for you.' This sounded quite mysterious.

'Sounds promising, Neil. I could be interested. You know Santos are after me for EM Queensland.'

'Yes, I have heard on the grapevine.' That was another of his attributes - he had ways of finding things out that I could only dream of. He was always ahead of the curve.

****

They flew me up and courted me at the Queensland Club. I was interviewed by the Chairman and Deputy Chairman of Crusader Oil on the personal recommendation of Neil. At the end of the meal they offered me the position of General Manager of Australian

Hydrocarbons. Crusader had secured a forty-nine percent controlling interest in Australian Hydrocarbons (AHY).

'You're only thirty-nine, aren't you?'

'That's correct,' I said.

'You'll be one of the youngest GM's in the country then. How's that sound?'

'Pretty good.'

'We expect you to consult back to Crusader on Cooper Basin Unit affairs, and work for Neil on those matters. Okay?'

'I understand. Leave it with me. I'll get back to you as soon as I discuss this with my wife. Thank you.'

****

Our six years in Melbourne had been happy ones. After twelve and a half years of married life with Kathy, I had converted to Catholicism in the progressive parish of Glen Waverley North at the Easter vigil of 1980. Father Hodges ran a welcoming church and gave meaningful and topical sermons. Accompanying Kathy and our children to Mass, I wanted to be more than an outside observer. I wanted to be a participant. The conversion was not the struggle that I, and undoubtedly most other observers, had anticipated. It was a subliminal, non-conscious moulding and acceptance as though some other was leading me. It was not something I tackled with my normal analytical scientific mind. There was a knowing, a natural completion of self. My life has been all the richer for that conversion. There had been no pressure from Kathy. It was her strong faith and her example that had brought me to this position. I thank her daily for her gift.

When I made the announcement to my parents, my father repeated his earlier words when I had announced I was marrying Kathy, 'Your grandfather will roll in his grave.'

I responded, 'Well that's good Dad at least he'll be facing the right way up again. He's been face down for a long while now.'

We had a house on a third of an acre in Vermont South that we loved. It was within close walking distance to the Morack Golf Club. The block was an unusual arrow shape at the end of a cul-de-sac and the house had been built on the point of the arrow with two backyards representing the barbs of that arrow. On one barb was the leisure space complete with swimming pool, and on the other barb we had a chook house, vegetable garden, and developing fruit trees. Kathy had developed her golfing passion and was the foundation Secretary/Treasurer of the Morack Ladies Golf Club. She had a rich group of friends and the girls were well established in their schools. We all enjoyed visiting Kathy's parents in Maryborough and following our struggling football side, Melbourne.

However, I had become a vagabond roamer forced initially upon me due to a strong survival instinct, but the roots can be traced back to the initial upheaval of my father's decision to move the family from Perth to Melbourne all those years ago. Moving was not the horror that so many around us make out, to us it had become a way of life. Some people hang on for an eternity but give up the opportunity to grow and experience new things. I knew no other way but mobility. I had learnt to be prepared to give stuff up in order to make way for new experiences and discoveries. Clean out the old, on with the new, keep moving. The soldier and the sniper know that a moving target is much harder to hit and go down, so keep moving while you can. As I set off for my eighteenth year as a geologist, Australian Hydrocarbons would be my eighth job. I was averaging less than three years per job, not exactly a stable life.

Kathy was left with yet another clean up, sale of house, and removal. I moved to commence my new position with Nicole and Suzie so that they could start in their new school, Loreto College in Coorparoo. It is not always easy gaining places in private schools that have waiting lists. I had obtained a reference from Father Hodges that was undoubtedly helpful. It attested to the fact that I was a good citizen and had served the parish school as Chairman of the Parents and Citizen's Council and President of the Netball Club. I was later to serve on the management committee of Loreto. I had been done over by the head nun, but we both knew that it was payback for the places that had been made for Nicole and Suzie in the school at such short notice.

The move was tough on Nicole as it was her last matriculation year of study. Kathy and Tess joined us several months later. Life was not meant to be easy.

60

METEORIC RISE AND RAPID FALL

Riding in the back seat of the taxi from the airport to the city, I was scanning a map of Brisbane when I asked the driver, 'What's this place Carindale? I don't know it.'

'It's a new suburb being developed by Suncorp,' the driver replied.

'Really? I like its location, easy access to the Gold and Sunshine coasts, and the airport.'

'Yeah, opened in 1980. Building a massive shopping centre out there now.'

'I'll take a look at it. I am moving up from Melbourne. I don't want to live out west again. I was in Jindalee years ago. If you live west of a city you are driving into the sun to go to work in the morning, and also coming home in the evening. I want to do something different this time.'

'Sounds like a good plan, man.'

I had negotiated AHY picking up three months accommodation as I looked for a home for the family. This was a far more sensible plan than the Aquitaine job. Perhaps I was maturing and getting smarter. I selected a flat on the corner of Albert and Charlotte Street in the heart of the city. I could run the girls to Loreto in the morning and they could catch the bus home in the afternoon. I could walk from the AHY/Crusader office at lunchtime. We developed a routine. I didn't have much idea of running a household to budget. We three would sit down to whole flounders and prawns. We were living like kings, but I needed Kathy to handle a budget. I had no understanding of freezing meals or cutting corners.

Kathy and Tess joined us towards the end of the three months, and we started house hunting in earnest. Kathy agreed with my decision that Carindale was a great option. The trouble was that most of the houses were two-story with little handkerchief sized backyards. They seemed claustrophobic compared with the third of an acre we had left in Melbourne. We upset the Suncorp real estate salesman so much with our indecision that he sheepishly approached me while Kathy was waiting in the back of his car and said, 'You could be interested in my house. It's got five bedrooms, three garages, a swimming pool on a quarter acre block, and is a single-story place at the end of a cul-de-sac. All the things you've been looking for. There is still some finishing off to do inside so you can make it your own.'

'Sounds good to me,' I replied.

'The only thing is you see, my wife doesn't know I want to sell it yet. Can you come on Sunday at ten o'clock when she's at church?'

We loved it as soon as we set foot in the door. It was on one of the biggest blocks in Carindale. It had a spacious yard and was a large rambling house ideal for a family. We agreed on a price.

'I'll just have to tell my wife now. I've over extended, I got these investment properties down the coast and I can't keep the show running, one of them has to go,' he said. My God, he's a braver man than me, I thought.

I described it as the house that fell off the back of a truck. We were to spend the next twenty-eight years in this house.

****

I was my own boss. My staff consisted of a personal secretary and a receptionist. The secretary was my choice, and one of the essential requirements was that she could take shorthand. I liked the power of dictating letters and other documents, there was something prime ministerial in that! I was running a publicly listed company with eleven million dollars in the bank, which was in several joint ventures, and I was reporting directly to the board. Because of the Crusader takeover of AHY I had inherited some very flash maroon leather furniture and desks from the AHY Sydney office of the pre-takeover Chairman, Sir Billy Sneddon. Crusader had organised some space on the floor above their offices in Creek Street for AHY. My father had reported to Billy Sneddon when he was Attorney General. He later rose to be Leader of the Opposition.

I did many things wrong as General Manager of Australian Hydrocarbons. I was enjoying benefits that were denied my compatriots within Crusader which was not conducive to having good relationships with them. I was separate and therefore an outsider. The setup was all wrong. They had given this young buck his head and I wanted to make something of Australian Hydrocarbons, not just be the lap dog of Crusader. I was required to report back to and serve Neil Gantry on Cooper Basin UTOC matters and attend monthly meetings with him in Adelaide. I preferred to be creating new business for AHY, seeking out farm-in (joint venture) opportunities and new exploration interests. I am aggressive and creative by nature, but not as sharp as I should be about the political ramifications involved.

The oil price fell to fourteen dollars a barrel in June 1986, and I was instructed by the board to "keep the powder dry," meaning reduce expenditure and to not be expansive. I had at that stage entered AHY into three new Surat Basin permits by way of farm-in. The other problem was I was reporting to a Claytons Chairman who took his instructions from the real power broker, the Chairman of Crusader. I repeatedly took a request to the board that I required a computer. Today, it sounds bizarre that I should have had to fight so hard to obtain a computer. The board never approved my computer and my continual requests just annoyed and aggravated them. The response was always, "keep the powder dry." I bought my own portable computer as I saw it to be essential for activities that I wished to pursue. It was a Sharp PC5000 that I carried around in a five-kilogram case the size of a *Singer* sewing machine, and it had one hundred and twenty-eight kilobytes of memory. This will sound even more bizarre to the modern reader.

My next mistake was to publicly disagree with the Chairman of Crusader while having a drink in a bar. I was called in by my Claytons Chairman on Friday morning to be told, 'Dennis, I have seen this all happen before. If it's between a director and staff, the director wins every time. There's not enough room in the company for you and the chairman.'

'I see.'

'The brash arrogance and defiance you displayed at the Club Bar on Wednesday may have been good for your ego, but let me tell you it had the opposite effect on the Chairman's ego. He has asked me to terminate your employment effective immediately.'

'I see.'

'I am sorry about this. It is not my decision. What are you going to do?'

I had to think quickly. If they thought I was going to retreat with my tail between my legs back to Melbourne they had another thing coming. 'I think I'll go consulting,' I replied.

'Good for you. I wish you well. I'll have a word to Gordon to make sure he throws some work your way.' Gordon was the Managing Director of Crusader,

'Well, thank you. That is most generous,' I managed through gritted teeth. I had learnt over the years to burn as few bridges as possible when it comes to the grand battle for survival.

****

That's the trouble with meteoric rises, they can be followed by a thudding fall. Kathy helped my flagging spirits by bravely remarking that I was maintaining my average employment at three years with a firm.

'I know you love your averages being the cricketer that you are,' she said.

"I would like this performance as a bowler, but as a batsman it's one lousy average.'

I received the call late in the afternoon of the Friday of the dismissal from Gordon. 'How would you like to come in on Monday? We have an idea and Neil and I would like to discuss a consulting opportunity with you,' Gordon said.

'Well thank you Gordon, I'll be in by nine o'clock.'

'Very well. See if you can have a good weekend.'

'Thanks,' I said before hanging up the phone.

****

Kathy and I had become tired of all these interstate moves, some self-inflicted but others forced due to the necessity of survival. As we were always on the move, we never quite felt like we belonged anywhere. Kathy had been a spartan putting up with all this turmoil and instability. She no doubt didn't expect this when she responded in the affirmative all those years ago to my question, 'How would you like to be married to a geologist?' She had become a good golfer playing pennant with the Brisbane Golf Club off a fourteen handicap. I joined her in social golf as best I could, but she would always manage to beat me. Once we were on the eighteenth green and I had a real chance to win. Her ball was further from the hole than mine and she was required to putt first. Before doing so she remarked, 'Do you realise if I sink this putt and you three putt from there I'll still beat you?'

'Go on,' I responded. Up until then the thought hadn't entered my head. Well she dropped a magnificent twenty-foot putt and I under pressure three putted from twelve feet. I took it on the chin as best I could with an extra drink at the nineteenth hole and further developed my ideas on Ian Chappell's sledging.

****

My entry into management had been brief. As I walked through Crusader's front door on the Monday morning following the dismissal, I saw it as a relaunch of my technical career as a geologist. I became the longest serving consultant operating in Brisbane, continuously serving Crusader as my sole client from Monday to Friday for eight years. I had extraordinary independence within a broad operating framework reporting to a talented Crusader triumvirate of Neil Gantry and the petroleum engineers, John Forrest and Tom Richman. Neil and John were particularly adroit on the legalistic interpretation of the documents that bound the Cooper Basin companies together, the operating agreement and the various joint venture agreements. Tom and I worked principally on the technical aspects. We were a strong team which would ultimately achieve much for Crusader, although Neil was to move on before the ultimate team triumph.

The Crusader Chairman was a distinguished entity around town which resulted in him having extended lunches at either the Queensland Club or the Brisbane Club, mixing in high powered circles. Because of these extended lunches he was not always on his game post lunch. For many years after my dismissal I would glimpse or hear the advance of the Chairman in the corridors of Crusader. He would pause at my office door and, looking in all bleary eyed towards me, must have caused confusion in his mind as he asked himself, 'I thought I dismissed that guy?' For my part, I did my best to hide behind my Singer sewing machine computer. I didn't invoice Crusader under my personal name but under my company name, so he wouldn't have seen my name through the accounts submitted to the board, and I had shaved my moustache off for good measure. I now wanted to look younger instead of older. Well, I escaped detection anyway.

61

HE GAVE US OUR VALUES
YOU KNOW

Early one morning in 1987, while GM of Australian Hydrocarbons, I received a call from my mother. At the age of seventy-four Dad had died in bed of a massive heart attack. I was overcome with sadness and guilt. I felt as though I had abandoned him in Perth. Why hadn't I given him more support when he needed it? The children heard the commotion and met me in the corridor.

'What's wrong Dad?' Suzie asked.

'Pa died last night,' and I hugged her as I uncontrollably cried.

On the flight over to Perth for the funeral, I would involuntarily cry as the memories of Dad's life returned to me. He had made so many sacrifices for his family to the detriment of his own happiness. He had met his problems and obstacles square on and always encouraged us to do the same. 'Don't worry about me son, you've got your own problems to look after,' he would quite often tell me. As I looked at him, now all reduced and small in his coffin, he surprised me as he had grown a beautiful grey-white beard and moustache. He had kept that a secret from me. It suited him and matched his thinning hair that had been neatly brushed straight back in the style he had used all his life. His hair had lost that tight crinkle and was now smooth, straight, and greatly thinned. But he looked peaceful, proud, handsome even. His own man at last, free.

I remarked to Brian as we looked at him, 'He gave us our values you know.' Brian quietly agreed and has remarked several times since then how those words had impacted on him. He was my beacon, my example of how to behave, meet life, and face adversity. Honour, fairness, sacrifice, all for family, hard work, courage, love, independence, were all gifts he had given by way of example. Encouragement enables, discouragement disables, and Dad had done nothing but encourage me in all my endeavours. 'You could be prime minister one day, son,' had been his constant mantra throughout my life. I had risen as far as I had on his encouragement, my attempt at not letting the side down. As I kissed him on the cheek in the coffin I told him that I loved him and whispered in his ear, 'Haven't made PM yet Dad, but made GM and sort of got close to your mate Billy Sneddon. I'll keep having a go.'

I had wanted to deliver a eulogy at the funeral or the wake, but an opportunity didn't arise. Aunt Joy and Brian did not provide the opportunity. That was a disappointment, but it is likely I would have been incapable of holding myself together. His rowing mates attended and that was a wonderful tribute and of course I caught up with Uncle Ted, Nev and Graeme, and other relatives. Aunt Eve had died years earlier. Mum was now without her partner. She insisted in staying in the family home but at least she had Aunt Joy, Uncle Ted, sisters, and some good neighbours that could look out for her. Brian in Canberra and myself in Brisbane were a long way away.

Mum passed away two and a half years later. After two years living independently in the family home it became evident that she could no longer stay there. We managed to place her in a nursing home. That wasn't easy. I had travelled to Perth to assist in the move only to be met with a resistant mother who had dug her heels in. She had changed her mind yet again, she didn't want to go. All my cajoling failed. I broke down on the phone to Brian, who had returned to Canberra. 'I don't know what to do with her. I can run drilling programs, budgets, and negotiate with a board of directors but Mum is too much. What do you think I should do?' He gave me wise counsel, 'Take your foot off the pedal. Give her the night in the house and then get some support from Joy and Aunt Dianne tomorrow. The three of you should be able to convince her it is the best thing for her.'

She died of stomach cancer. It had spread to such an extent that it was inoperable. Aunt Joy and Brian were with her at the end. I selfishly was too busy in Brisbane trying to hold my own family and career together as a self-employed consultant. My heart was not torn in the same way over Mum's death as my father's. That's a very sad thing to say as I write these words, but there had been so much to overcome. The pain of abandonment at the age of thirteen, the confused messages of smothering love intermingled with absences and periods of insanity had left an indelible imprint on my heart and psyche. It had resulted in a barrier between us that became impenetrable. I can say no more on this, I feel empty. I know she tried. I now have the maturity to know that everyone in their own way, to their own capacity, gives of themselves as best they can. I have written in the earlier chapters the great gifts she gave me, and I am eternally grateful. Mum, I live my life honouring your sacrifices as well.

62

A DASH AT POLITICS

Before discussing my time as a consultant with Crusader it is necessary to explain some of my other activities while General Manager of Australian Hydrocarbons. My career up until that point had been solely dominated by developing my technical skills. So many of my years had been spent on fieldwork talking to the trees. How was I to compete and communicate with the Michelle Frydenbergs of this world? I became active in Rostrum to gain confidence as a public speaker. Also, I had been invited to join the Liberal Party. I became a very active member and held various positions in the party: Secretary, Chairman, Treasurer, and Social Secretary of the Creek Road Branch.

Moving into management required me to learn to read a balance sheet, so I enrolled in the Securities Institute of Australia Diploma in Applied Finance and Investment, and I was granted that qualification in 1992. It is well regarded, and I flirted with the idea of being either an investment analyst or personal financial planner. My work history and the insecurity of employment as a geologist was the main driver to being fleet footed and developing alternative options.

Another option was to enter politics. Maybe I could indeed be prime minister one day as my father had continually encouraged. I gained experience working on several campaigns. I assisted on polling day which resulted in the election of Brian Taylor in the 1988 Groom by-election. Also in 1988 I was Chairman of the Carina Campaign Committee for the seat of Chatsworth and celebrated the election of Graeme McDougall. The seat was retained in 1991 despite being held by only a one and a half percent margin. It was a thrilling campaign triumph. I ran for pre-selection twice, once for the state seat of Mansfield and once for the federal seat of Moreton. Neither time was I selected as the candidate. Moreton was held by Labor with the thin margin of two percent, and it was hotly contested by quality candidates. Margaret Stein, a lawyer, won the nomination. I still had a way to go. Maybe I had been talking to trees for too long but Dad, I gave it a go.

I wanted to be involved with the John Hewson run at the prime ministership. I believed in the bravery of the man and his manifesto, *Fightback,* the boldest detailed reform package ever put out by an Opposition Leader to the Australian public. He was defeated by the most brutal sledger in Australian politics, Paul Keating. One of the best and most equitable tax initiatives for Australia, the GST, was to be denied the Australian public for another six years, until the Howard government introduced it in 1999.

Analysts have attributed Hewson's defeat to his response to reporter Mike Willesee's question on the GST payable on a birthday cake. From that point forth the complicated game of cat and mouse between journalists and politicians has intensified such that intelligent discussion of matters of substance has become almost impossible. Journalists in search of 'got-you' moments and politicians 'playing the backward defensive stroke'. It's an unfair contest and much to the detriment of Australia.

My own manifesto for the pre-selection was a document I provided to delegates that highlighted my attributes and vision for Australia. It read,

'I believe in a strong, vigorous, growing Australia that provides wealth, promise, opportunity and security for present and future generations of Australians.'

Does the average Australian understand the effort required to have a run at politics? The number of branch meetings that the candidate attends and at which speeches are made? The mindless fundraising events that are required to be organised? I put on a dedicated research assistant to write speeches and articles for newspapers to lift my profile. I personally spent a minimum of five thousand dollars on the campaign for pre-selection, only to lose. I figured I could manage it while the consulting income was coming in.

I am convinced that people enter politics for all the right reasons. They want to make a difference and a positive contribution, but it is an exhausting, thankless task that sucks the energy out of you, and it ultimately defeats most. I received wonderful support from the Creek Road branch, Senator Warwick Parer and his wife Kathy, and Don Cameron, who had held the seat of Moreton after taking over from Sir Jim Killen.

Events out of my control would soon take over our lives, and active political involvement was to abruptly cease. It became the least of my concerns.

63

DAVID OVER GOLIATH VICTORY

The UTOC 1/1/87 Review and Adjustment was never completed due to the Crusader team of which I was a part. The gas flowing from the Moomba processing plant of the South Australian Cooper Basin Gas Unit provided both Sydney and Adelaide's gas supply.

Neil Gantry had set the scene through early battles over the geologic mapping of gas in place, especially in the mapping of the zero line. Neil eventually left Crusader for greener pastures, and the overall direction of our effort passed to John Forrest.

As a team we studied all the legal agreements binding the Cooper Basin joint venturers together and we understood the key drivers that determined equity distribution. My history of working with small companies was invaluable. In a small company there is nowhere to hide. All members must carry their own weight and then some. I had been required to review all legal documents while serving both Beach and Alliance.

The thrust of the team was that Crusader was being disadvantaged by the methods of calculation of both the hydrocarbons in place and the recoverable reserves within the unitised Cooper Basin fields. Crusader gas fields were of a far superior reservoir quality when compared to the other producing companies. Applying the same statistically based calculation methods across all fields, regardless of their reservoir quality, was inequitable. This flowed through to the participation factors of each company and their ultimate revenue.

John's father had been a politician. This meant that he had been raised in a house exposed to political debate all his life. He had an acerbic tongue and a quick mind. When he spoke, all would listen. He could command a room like Paul Keating. A leader exudes confidence in many ways. They need to stand apart, be slightly aloof, and not just one of the boys. They have an all-knowing air or at least a bit of mystery that they have knowledge beyond your own as a mere follower. Through that confidence they display a courage and ruthlessness that followers alone do not have. John had all those qualities.

Tom and I were more like street fighters, both raised in the hurly burly of state schools with no private school handshake behind which to hide. John had class; we had grit, staying power, and determination. Together we were a team to take to the trenches. We were convinced of the righteousness of our cause, saw it as a war, and fought accordingly.

Our battle ground was technical purity and correctness. Our goal was to restore equity between the Joint Venture partners' revenue stream and secure Crusader its rightful pay cheque. Match day for us was the once a month UTOC meetings held in Adelaide. I had already become an experienced hand at attending these meetings, having done so for three years as an Alliance representative and three years while GM of Australian Hydrocarbons. This would be my arena for the next eight years, but the most dramatic act of all would be the first three years climaxing in a court case against Santos as Operator.

We were a mix of detective, journalist, politician, and soldier. Large companies and government departments grow to a level of slovenly obesity in which all members of the organisation are not a tight unit. There is always disunity within the protective employment umbrella, and they do not all support each other. Petty jealousies abound. There is a scramble to gain the next important promotional title and some practise actively undermining colleagues to advance. The level of command is long and tortuous, and internal communication is fragmented.

In large companies the biggest drain on productivity is endless meetings. The brightest become managers who become less and less productive as they delegate to underlings. The manager's life becomes one of attending meetings such that they are not doing any real work and are merely conducting reviews. So instead of the best brains working on the problem, the work is conducted by the less experienced. Also, the underling is less than enthusiastic as he has been instructed by the 'manager' as to how it should be done. He is not given his head to develop his own methodology and creativity to solve the problem. What results is low morale for both the manager and worker.

This is not a problem in a small team. A small team is vibrantly alive and has fun in the process. If you are the only geologist on the team, what does it matter if you are the Chief Geologist or the Junior Geologist, you are the geologist and guess what: you do the geology because there is no other. You cannot delegate, you do it yourself and make discoveries in the process. Innovative ideas germinate not in a prescribed rigid framework or to a tight timetable. Individuals solve problems and create fresh solutions, not committees and large organisations. It is well known in the resources industries that individuals and small companies make the breakthrough discoveries. Then they become a part of history as large companies take them over and manage those discoveries. That is the normal cycle.

Small companies are more dynamic and flexible. Errors and dead-end theories are abandoned once tested. There are no departments or manager egos that need protection. Our focus and unity would ultimately win out.

The Unit had developed gas in place mapping techniques that I could question and a petrophysics equation, the Overton equation, that was indiscriminately run over all the reservoirs to determine the quantity of gas in place. It was based on, and a revision of, an earlier equation, the Porter equation, developed by a leading Australian petrophysicist Chris Porter. The equation had served its purpose as a 'ready reckoner' in the early days of exploration of the Cooper Basin. As a cost cutting exercise, the basin developed with the dominant, and in most cases the only, porosity tool run in so many wells being the sonic log. Porosity is a term which refers to the pore space in a rock, which is the holding capacity of the fluids, whether those fluids be gas, oil or water. It is a basic and fundamental parameter to be determined.

The most recognised determination of porosity uses the Wyllie time average equation. I analysed the Wyllie equation to death. The Porter and Overton equations suffered due to their statistical averaging. I refined the application of the Wyllie equation to the different fields in order to honour the varying input parameters to the equation which were temperature, depth of burial, and zone dependent. I conducted much of my log analysis on my Singer sewing machine portable computer using elaborate spreadsheets established from first principles. I would look at the sensitivities of changing the input parameters to the output results. Once I had achieved this I could then compare my results to those of the Operator using the Overton equation.

Anomalies and trends soon became evident. Crusader was missing out on revenue due to the application of the Overton equation. Other companies were getting their unfair share of reserves and revenue.

Tom and I worked together closely. Given his head, he reviewed the intricacies of reservoir engineering which control the recovery of hydrocarbons from the gas in place, chief amongst which is permeability. We shared adjacent offices, so our interchange was frequent, immediate and on demand as much as required. Try doing that in a big company!

I provided Tom with the geologic and petrophysical front end to reservoir model runs that he would perform. These runs would produce production profiles and a predicted ultimate recovery of gas or reserves. The reliability of the reservoir model is determined from what is called - history matching. For a mature producing field, this can be graphically displayed by overlaying actual production to model forecast production. The better the history match the assumption is the better, the truer, the more reliable, the most representative, the model. If you play with these models, however, you begin to realise that the solutions are not unique. Matching can be achieved with a tweak here, a tweak there, and an altered assumption. So much geologic detail is lost in the required 'upscaling' of getting the data into the model which begs the question: where is the truth?

****

The technical battles were fierce and not for the faint hearted. One Santos presenter came up with an amusing statement when in debate, 'You guys are micro-metering the watermelon.' In other words, we were being pedantic, and our arguments on fine detail probably didn't change the size of the reserves. Of course, that was something we vehemently denied. Our very existence depended upon highlighting those differences. Santos cycled through managers to chair the UTOC meetings in the hope that they could turn the tide against the Crusader assault. It was a poisoned chalice appointment for any of their managers as we were in the ascendancy.

My petrophysical attacks were beginning to bite, so much so that it came to a head at one UTOC meeting. Santos brought to the meeting the two leading petrophysicists in Australia at that time, Chris Porter and Hugh Crocker. They were there to defend their position and support the veracity of applying the Overton equation to determine porosity. I, very much the generalist, traded blows with them. It takes courage to publicly disagree with specialists in front of your peers, but I managed to hold my own under fire. One of the greatest tributes I received many years later, as I was dining in the Santos mess hall, came from the then Santos Chief Petrophysicist. He said, 'I think you should know that you were quite right in that dispute over the Overton equation.' That meant a great deal to me as he was a very experienced petrophysicist from an international company who had come to Santos after the dispute and had reviewed the minutes of all the meetings.

****

Crusader had such faith in our technical case that they took Santos to court over the 1/1/87 Review and Adjustment. The case was heard in the Supreme Court of South Australia. John, Tom, and I flew to Adelaide. Crusader was represented by barristers and a Queens Council. Legal cases involve a lot of paper. We would work late at night in the legal firm's office, and their large photocopiers hummed along as we held strategy meetings. Dependent upon how the proceedings had gone during the day, after debriefing and review, the strategy could change. There was an adrenalin rush in being involved in such a high-stakes game. Fortunately, Tom and

I were not required to take the stand, but our leader John had to take the full brunt of cross examination from the Santos lawyers. He acquitted himself well.

After ten days Judge Bollen ruled in favour of Santos. Undeterred, Crusader felt there were errors of judgement in the decision by the S.A. judge and quickly made an appeal to the Australian High Court. Approximately a year following the initial judgement in S.A. the five High Court judges ruled three to two in favour of Crusader. We had finally won. As a result, Santos had to pay all Crusader's legal fees and reached a settlement which included an ex gratia payment of tens of millions of dollars and an adjusted fixed participation factor locking in a significant revenue gain. We were ecstatic and celebrated appropriately.

My celebration was to be short lived however. I was about to face my biggest challenge as a human being.

PART 4 -
MATURITY
1991 – 2016

"Even our troubles and our heartbreaks tell us something about our true destiny"
John Eldredge

64

IT CAN ALL CHANGE IN A MOMENT

1991 was our annus horribilis. Sinatra's words, *"Riding high in April, shot down in May"* come so easily to mind, just change the months to November and December.

The blood clot was on a mission – search and destroy. It was lazy on the search but diligent, effective with the 'destroy'. It doesn't matter what is destroyed – the military call it 'collateral damage.' Devoid of consciousness, it indiscriminately snuffs out whatever lies before it. The clot was released from a heart in trouble with a leaky mitral valve. We were told it was a consequence of the rheumatic fever she had as a child. Carried by the life-giving oxygenated blood, the clot advanced along the cerebral artery. As the blood vessels narrowed, the clot would hang up occasionally on the arterioles but still flow on. Like a narrowing pipe, the distribution network takes the blood and the clot ever forward until finally bam, the capillary is too narrow - it can advance no further. Downstream of the blockage the brain is starved of oxygen, denied of life, and neurotransmitters fail.

Kathy had just stepped out of the shower and was towelling off when the bam occurred. She tried to brace her fall by making a grab for the towel rail, but it was to no avail. She dropped to the floor. I heard her fall and raced to the bathroom. I called out her name, but she could not respond; she couldn't speak. I sat her up as best I could. She was of normal weight but a person in collapse is a dead weight. I would need another person to assist me. I rang our GP. He was there quickly. He confirmed what I feared, she had suffered a stroke. He rang for an ambulance. She was taken to the Mater hospital with the doctor and me following. She received immediate attention. From what I now know, I should have rung the ambulance myself. It would have saved precious minutes and it is so important to act fast to limit the brain damage.

Just over twenty-four hours earlier she was enjoying herself with her golf friends at their Christmas break up party, telling jokes like she always loved to do. It was Friday the 13th, a portent of what was to come perhaps? The event, the bam occurred at 7.00pm on Saturday the 14th December 1991. It is a date and time we will never forget. We had been married for twenty-four years at that stage, she just forty-seven and me forty-five years old. It is a date that marks pre- and post-stroke existence, the before and the after, the dividing line between what might have been and what is reality. It is now another twenty-six years on and maybe the symmetry is appropriate for me to write this reflection now. In that instant our lives were transformed.

She was propped up in bed the next day, paralysed down the right side, face drooping down, incapable of speech. The doctors assured me they had done and were doing all that they could. It had been a left-brain stroke and had affected her speech centre. She had lost the swallow reflex, so she was being fed through a drip.

Pain comes dressed in all sorts of different clothes. It is the powerlessness that really hurts. Suzie and I left her on the Sunday to attend evening Mass in search of solace, in search of meaning. I quietly wept and sobbed as the hymnal words were sung,

Will you live with me the darkness as I die?

We had looked into the abyss and saw, felt, fear and death. Dread of the future that lay ahead. I wept then and I weep still but my God I love her deeply. Her courage is boundless.

Ambition quickly turns to survival. I had the ambition to be a politician. Given the state of politics today it sounds so comical now - aspiring to be a politician. It is such a brutal game, a destructive and thankless game. I had seen enough destruction. I was witnessing real physical and mental destruction with my wife. It was clear where my responsibilities lay from this time forward and it was certainly not with the selfish, ego driven pursuit of politics. All my energies were with her recovery and the preservation of our family. I had the wonderful example of my father who had faced many family crises. You press on, laugh at adversity, and spit in its face.

It's like a mugging. Without invitation and without choice, Kathy had been robbed of so much. She had done the hard yards raising our three children. Nicole had just married in the September, Suzie just graduated with a university degree, and only I could attend that proud occasion as Kathy was in hospital. Only Tess, with two years of secondary schooling, remained to nurture into the future. I had seen the green shoots of Kathy's blossoming be prematurely cut. Her reward for years of mothering, the promise of something else, all denied to her because of the unwanted December 14th 'clot' visitor.

Now we had to face the fight back, reclaim life. She was allowed home on New Year's Day. She had recovered from most of her right-side paralysis but needed occupational therapy to reclaim many of the necessary functionalities. Right-side muscular weakness would remain with her for the rest of her life. She was suffering from dyspraxia and dysphasia, and would need speech therapy for over two years to recover the ability to speak. This was a complete relearning, a rewiring of neurotransmitters with the establishment of new pathways in the brain. Kathy is a courageous fighter and determinedly tackled her recovery. Pre-stroke she was a good golfer playing off a fourteen handicap. Part of her rehabilitation was to bring her back to golf. She received great support from her golfing mates. It was a hard path however and it became less satisfying for her when she could not even play to a thirty-six handicap. The inability to add up the card, another deficit caused by the stroke, ultimately became too embarrassing despite the protestations of her mates. She finally discarded that great passion as a bad joke.

Our whole mode of socialising changed overnight. I became the organiser and the chief spokesman for us. She had been the primary socialiser before. It was a reversal of roles. The truth is that you never quite get over a stroke and what you have lost. I said to her once that it took me at least ten years to get over her stroke. She said make that fifteen for me. She was an avid reader. She still reads but it is so much harder for her, and it takes her four weeks to read what she may have read in one week.

Life involves a daily death and a daily rise. It is won through struggle, not submission, but the struggle has to be informed and with an understanding that at times you must accept and go with the flow. Kathy's biggest deficit has been her speech. She has come a long way, and we now know how to communicate with each other. I understand her so well I intuitively know where she is heading with her thoughts and speech, however, in mixed company she is so often forced to take on the role of passive listener.

We have moved on now. She loves the theatre, ballet, musicals, TV, plays a mean game of five hundred, the Brisbane Lions and Aussie Rules, tennis and cricket on TV, going over to Stradbroke Island, and travel. She loves cooking meals for me too! We are doing one overseas trip a year while we have the health to do so. Once that gets too difficult we'll convert to domestic only (Postscript: by 2016 it became too hard, just domestic now).

I want to hug and embrace her, envelop her in my arms, to be her protector, her saviour, put her back together again. Like Humpty Dumpty though, that's just not possible. Sometimes I hug her too tight and she can't breathe, the emotions too overwhelming. Could I have done more? That is a trip you are always on. At the hour of the test, did I do okay? They are all questions without answers.

65

I KNEW I HAD LOST
MY BEST MATE

These years were dark; I was besieged by sadness and trauma. I had kept in touch with Dave Slipper, my best friend from my schooldays and my best man at our wedding. Always working in retail, his goal was to run his own business one day. Another of his early dreams was to get his pilot's licence, a dream befitting his daredevil courage and Clarke Gable swagger through life, which was of course one of his endearing qualities. He had married the beautiful livewire girl Rochelle and they had three children, Matthew, Craig, and Chloe. They had lived in Launceston, Melbourne, Morwell, and then Port Macquarie cycling through many small business operations like news agency, sandwich bar, and delicatessen.

Dave achieved his dream by owning a sporting store in Port Macquarie. This was heaven for first class Dave that only wanted the best in sporting gear. He could get all the best at wholesale prices as a shop owner. He sold guns, rode his Bugatti around town, and could live out his wild adventurous dreams. Rochelle worked at the TAFE in some administrative capacity. The two of them were well loved entities in Port Macquarie with a full social life. I also became close to Matthew. He was studying at the University of Queensland, and he would help me out on Saturday mornings to maintain the large backyard of our Carindale house. He was a good worker, very courteous and had developed his father's taste for riding motor bikes. The whole court knew when Matthew had arrived to start work with me.

On our last annual visit to see the Slippers, I could see things were not altogether right with their middle son Craig. He had the moroseness of the lost soul and the clipped-on eye balls of the drug addict of which I had been exposed to at the iron ore mine all those years back. Dave and Rochelle told me stories of him being delivered home to them in police cars. Because they were so well respected and loved in the community the police were more tolerant of Craig's indiscretions than they might have been with any other person. He had been given many chances so that he could avoid the disgrace of obtaining a police record.

It had become a great concern to them. 'It's like he just wants to fail,' Dave said. 'We don't know what to do with him. I managed to get him a job helping a mate of mine doing tiling.'

'How did he go?' I asked.

'He's not reliable. When he's clean his work is very good, but then he goes missing.'

'Shame.' I could see the pain in his eyes and the depth of hopelessness in my friend's heart.

'I'll give you an example of his self-sabotaging, bizarre behaviour. Rotary had organised a fundraising charity event which involved a ten-kilometre run along the beach in heavy sand. Craig was a hundred yards ahead of the pack with the finish line in sight when he just decided to stop. He sat down on a rock with this stupid smile on his face, and when the last runner had passed him he got up and ran to the line.'

'Bloody crazy. What was that all about?'

'I guess he was trying to say, look I can easily beat you guys, but this doesn't mean a thing to me. It was like thumbing his nose up at the lot of us. Stuff the lot of you, you are the crazy ones.'

'Jesus, I don't know what to say.' The conversation ended as we gazed into our beers. It was the gaze of incomprehension as many things just cannot be understood.

****

The day following this discussion Dave, Matthew, Craig, one of their next-door neighbours and I drove to the beach for a swim. It was a bad plan because it was a wild day. The seas were huge with violent near shore dumping waves and aggressive rips. Dave had always challenged me with his escapades. I would follow him into the trenches, so I gave him the benefit of the doubt and I entered the water only to be brutally dumped near the shore. I felt the power of the undertow and I knew this wasn't for me. I was the first to get out of the water and only a brief time after the others followed, all except Craig.

'Where the hell is Craig?' Dave asked. We all gazed seaward, fearing the worst. The minutes ticked on.

'There he is, right out there,' said Matthew. He was a good three hundred metres away.

'Bloody fool. What's he doing right out there?' Dave was greatly relieved but grim lipped. He waved furiously at him to come back to shore but Craig either didn't see us, didn't care, or had other plans. Good friends can read each other's thoughts, and I knew what was going through Dave's mind.

After a good fifteen minutes had transpired Craig turned and half swam, half surfed to shore. Exhausted, he collapsed on the beach claiming he had been caught in a rip and decided it was best not to fight it but let it carry him out until he could escape it. This was a plausible explanation in hindsight, but was there the scent of a near miss suicide on the salty sea breeze?

****

Back in Brisbane, we were watching the news after our evening meal when the story broke. I knew I had lost my best mate. It was a tragedy. 'Family slaughtered in Port Macquarie, only one survivor, son detained and been taken to the Kempsey gaol,' the reporter announced. 'The deranged son was discovered still with knife in hand the next day.'

He had killed his brother downstairs while he was in bed sleeping. Matthew had no chance. Dave, hearing the racket, had descended from his upstairs bedroom and was ambushed at the base of the stairs. Rochelle's body was found at the top of the stairs. Chloe had escaped as she no longer lived at home.

At the funeral the heavy air of disbelief and incomprehension that these beautiful people had lost their lives in such a horrible way hung in the church. I hugged Chloe to my chest and mumbled some words, 'I am so sorry, Chloe. He was my best mate.'

She was so stoic, she simply replied, 'I know.'

'If there is anything I can do, please call.'

'Yes,' she replied as we continued to hug.

What life is ahead for Craig, incarcerated for life because of a moment of drug- induced insanity? His is an example of marihuana-induced schizophrenia on a young developing brain. What nightmares lie ahead for Chloe? She lost her family overnight.

66

MID LIFE CRISIS

These years were my midlife crisis years. I was lost, emotionally alone, distraught, and trying my best to cope. Keep the flag flying, keep the boat afloat, like a Dutchman plug up the holes in the dyke: all sound like such shallow metaphors. I would have drowned if it was not for the compassion of John Forrest and Tom Richman. I had proven my mettle with the Santos court case victory, but they kept me on well beyond my use-by date. As a result, our personal plight was not compounded by financial ruin as well. In fact, quite the opposite; the eight years of continual consultancy with them helped secure our financial future.

I started researching how I could assist my beautiful wife's recovery. I had started learning Tai Chi some years prior and loved the calming influence that it had on my stress levels. I took both Kathy and Tess to classes. Tess took to it very well and it is a passion of hers to this very day. It was not to Kathy's liking, however. A friend had started teaching Feldenkrais. Kathy and I started lessons with him. Feldenkrais is all to do with movement, how we move, the efficiency of movement and how we can adapt ourselves to move differently, particularly after some trauma. It was an interesting health modality which we pursued for over a year.

I continued with my Tai Chi. I had become fascinated by the Chinese health model and its accompanying philosophy. It gave me insight into what had happened to our family. I was reading alternative health books and mind-body books. I was reading about how cancer sufferers had overcome their illness. The power of the mind and the interweaving web of physical, emotional, and spiritual pathways to good health emerged from my readings. I decided to enrol at the College of Natural Medicine in Spring Hill to study acupuncture. I adjusted my consulting hours with Crusader to attend lectures and practicals.

I needed to slow down to find my centre - not an easy task for a hyperactive personality like mine. I started a daily journal not only to record what was happening within my family and their progress back to health, but to help me process these changes in my life. The journal proved to be invaluable. I was living through the non-acceptance phase with the belief that if I search and struggle hard enough I will find a solution.

My friendship with my Feldenkrais friend developed. He was struggling with the intractable problem of having employment in Brisbane and a girlfriend in Sydney. He was also exploring avenues of personal development. We embarked together on some very advanced Qigong methods under Master Jirong Zhang. My friend boarded for a month with us in our large Carindale house at a time when he was changing houses. We would arise at day break and practice our reverse abdominal breathing in the horse stance with arms extended horizontally out to the side at shoulder height, receiving the universal energy. We built up slowly until we were both managing ninety minutes in this stance. Muscle fatigue would set in and they would twitch and vibrate.

There were two techniques that assisted in maintaining this practice for ninety minutes. One was always returning to the reverse abdominal breathing and visualising the intake of energy from the sun and heavens above through the hands, and the energy from Mother Earth through the feet. The other, which I found to be the most powerful, was imagining all my ancestors, family, and friends holding my arms up. The arms become very heavy after being held out for all that time. So, while maintaining the breathing, our individual support teams would be mentally dragged in to assist one at a time. This was a powerful technique that induced a daily connection with, and acknowledgement of, all the people who had brought you to this point in your life and those who were now in your life. The interweaving and interdependence of all, to the good health of all, is then understood and appreciated.

Despite all these personal development efforts, I still had not learnt the go-slow technique to good health very well. I had difficulty letting life just happen; solutions will emerge if only you would trust in the universe. I had to keep trying and forcing it along. In parallel with the Natural Medicine Institute studies, I started a faster track to becoming an acupuncturist by doing other studies with Geoff Wilson at The Traditional Healing Arts Centre. Geoff taught Daoist philosophy and put me in touch with understanding the patient's illness at the deepest emotional level. To get to the core of a patient's problem demands superior counselling skills. The right questions need to be asked, and the responses listened to and completely understood with the right level of compassion. It requires great skill. It cannot be done unless you, the healer, are at peace with yourself and have dealt with all of your own demons. Geoff Wilson's Barefoot Doctor course provided deeper insight to healing than the more conventional diploma that I would have received from the Institute. To be any good, I needed both.

I rushed into opening an acupuncture clinic, and I rented some space above Wallace Bishop's in the Queen Street Mall in Brisbane. By now I had acquired a useful craft. I could do Shiatsu chair massages to a good standard and with a set routine. I was a pseudo-acupuncturist, practicing without a recognised qualification and no insurance. In conducting chair massages, I would sometimes go in too hard on pressure points, and I could lose clients fainting due to blood pressure changes in their body. I would have to revive them with a rescue formula or smelling salts. I helped one lady to the floor as she was violently ill into a waste paper bin held between her legs. After she recovered, I escorted her down the mall to a taxi. She didn't return. This incident frightened the life out of me, and I decided to shut down the clinic.

I was putting our financial future at risk. I was conducting Shiatsu chair massages at weekend markets. On a good day I could make one hundred dollars. With great pride I would come home, put the money on the table and say to Kathy, 'There you are love, good quality pot roast this week.' This was not at all fair to Kathy. She was having her own struggle in processing her way through her stroke recovery, and here was her husband going off the deep end with change of life experimentations into Qigong practices and alternative therapies.

Not totally off the rails just yet, I attempted some alternate income by selling off our share portfolio. The portfolio was performing very well. In a rising market I became a ten percent trader. That is realising profits through sale when the stock had risen by that amount. It was a simple formula and in a rising market quite foolproof. I ignored the maxim that whenever anything is going well don't change it. I shut down the portfolio, and we invested one hundred and fifty thousand dollars in a brick works at Kleinton, near Toowoomba. The plan was that this would provide an independent income stream through dividends. At the time of investment, the company had forty-five percent of the Toowoomba brick market. We received one dividend; the general manager resigned and took a lot of business with him, and then the impact of a long drought dampened Toowoomba growth. The investors scrambled to keep the place afloat, but over a protracted period we parted with our one hundred and fifty thousand dollars.

I had lost a smaller amount of five thousand dollars over the acupuncture clinic exercise. It could have been a lot more. Wallace Bishop had me over a barrel in a rental agreement but compassionately released me from the contract. But as they say in advertising, there's more. I had befriended a fellow student, Ah So, at the Natural Medicine Institute. He was a much younger man than I as well as a Qigong and martial arts enthusiast. He had several business concepts. The first was to buy a *'Walk Safe'* franchise. *'Walk Safe'* was a self-defence technique developed to ward off aggressors. We travelled to Sydney together in my car so Ah So could meet and be trained in the technique by the franchisors. The franchisors worked in some sleazy back alley alongside a building flashing a purple neon sign, *'Tilleys.'* I soon worked out what sort of business that was. I was feeling quite uncomfortable as the boys would work out whizzing their Philippine fighting sticks within an inch of doing extreme damage to anyone and sundry.

Ah So's other idea was to get into fight promotions and martial arts demonstrations involving overseas exponents. Desperate times require desperate actions, so I was considering everything and anything, but the reality was that I hadn't made a good call for quite some time now. All I could see was another money drain in a risky venture. I had to say no to Ah So and shut down our business partnership. I had been providing all the seed capital to these ventures. I had just burnt up another five thousand dollars.

I had to stop this money drain, so I put the muscle onto Ah So to come up with some work for me.

67

BIG JO JO HOHEPA

And so, here I was ringside about to watch the Australasian Kick Boxing Championship title bout at the Redcliffe Hotel. I could not remember the last time I had made a good decision. Ah So had arranged this gig for me to massage one of the boxers.

I was not fully trained in massage; I was a fledgling in the craft, but I knew that you could either stimulate or relax through massage depending on technique. Tonify or sedate. I was wheeled in to meet big Jo Jo Hohepa and when I saw him, all memory of my miniscule training instantly evaporated. Jo Jo was massive, a front row forward to frighten front row forwards. His head had an unusual vertical taper to it and had been shaven to prickly black fuzz. His face and arms were ornamented with Ta Moko traditional Maori tattoos. This man had ancestral roots that I would never understand. He was stripped to the waist and had boxer shorts around his loins. This guy was a heavy weight. I, more so now because of my sleepless nights, was bantam weight, a mere sixty-five kilograms, half the fighter's weight. My eyes were drawn to Hohepa's massive biceps, and I was overcome with the thought that it would be impossible for even both my hands to encircle them. Raw fear rose up within me, a taste of bile in the throat, and a loose feeling in the bowels. This all happened before a word was spoken. I managed to pull myself together and as confidently as my remaining courage allowed asked,

'So Jo Jo, what sort of massage do you want from me, Swedish, Oriental, Chinese, Shiatsu, Sports? I can do the lot you know. Been round the footy clubs doing this stuff for years,' I lied.

'Just do your stuff then, man. Leave it to you. You've got an hour,' was all that Hohepa said. And with that, he mounted the massage table and lay on his stomach. Even from this brief encounter, I observed that Hohepa was already in the zone. His eyes exuded an intense calm in the knowledge of his need to do battle, and maybe the resignation of the possible pain to come. As I was massaging I imagined what was going through Hohepa's mind. Was he thinking of ring craft strategy, technique, or was he a warrior thinking of glory?

This was the biggest massage job I had ever had. Going through my mind was, *Don't stuff this up. Make a mistake and you could be scrambled eggs for Hohepa's breakfast. Where is Ah So? I've been left alone in this room with Hohepa.*

Fortunately, the Maori warrior in his pre-match preparation was not on for a talk, a man of few words, so I was free to wholly concentrate on my technique. I was observing muscles that I had only read about. The resistance coming back from these muscles was sucking the energy out of me. Even with the best of technique and application, I could not penetrate with any depth through the tight, firm layers.

I concentrated hard and poured myself into my work. His sweat and my sweat mixed with the oils I was applying. The Maori's arms must have weighed six kilograms, and I was continually lifting them up, drawing them behind his back and placing them down again. I was totally exhausted when Ah So appeared and announced, 'Hour's up you two. Time to get ready Jo Jo.'

Jo Jo rose from the table and looked me in the eye. 'Good massage, man. You fix him up Ah So.'

'Sure.'

The two left the room and I packed up my gear. I thought Hohepa's eyes were beyond an intense calm. He looked down right sleepy. I hoped I had done the right thing.

****

Fully spent, I took up my reserved front row, ringside seat. It was an oppressively humid evening in mid-February. I looked around the crowd. It was obvious that many of them had been there in the bars, drinking all day. The overpowering smell of stale beer mixed with dry cigarette smoke. This crowd had been waiting for a long-time, thirsty for blood and eagerly anticipating the brutality to come.

A roar went up as the two fighters entered the ring. Killer Bazza was Hohepa's opponent, a redneck from the deep south of the US. He was slightly smaller than Big Jo but maybe that would aid his speed. The referee gave the compulsory instructions to fight fair. Bit of a joke of course, as almost anything is allowed in kick boxing.

Killer Bazza came out blazing and pushed Big Jo into a corner. Jo was defending as best he could, carefully deflecting brutal kicks. Big Jo looked slow, sluggish and without energy. I was thinking, *Oh no. I've gone and sedated him instead of tonified him. This is entirely my fault. I could be in big trouble with Ah So and the fight promoters.*

Big Jo survived the first round. It all happened again though in the second round. Killer throwing everything at Big Jo with the Maori just fending off attacks and absorbing what managed to get through his defence. My anxiety was mounting. This same pattern went on for seven rounds. I was looking around to see where I could quickly exit in order to save my own skin.

Just before the start of the eighth round, Big Jo looked straight at me and, with a little sideways movement of his head, winked. With false swagger I winked back. He struck his right fist into the palm of his left hand and in response I yelled, 'Go get him, big fella!'

Both myself and the crowd had totally underestimated Hohepa. The big fella had been playing rope-a-dope with Killer. Killer had exhausted himself with outright attacks while Big Jo had been conserving his energy. Big Jo gave Killer a massive kick in the lower leg which almost floored him. The fight was over at that point, but Big Jo toyed with him a bit more before finishing him off late in the ninth.

After the speeches and presentation, Ah So jumped into the ring and triumphantly escorted Big Jo back to the rooms. For a moment, I contemplated going back stage to ask for a bonus, but common sense prevailed, and I went out the nearest exit, grateful to be alive. I drove home wondering had Hohepa just implemented his premeditated strategy or had it taken him seven rounds to get over my sedating massage?

68

LIKE FINE WINE A GEOLOGIST MATURES

My midlife crisis served a purpose. It had put me in touch with my inner self. All the setbacks as I stumbled forward had provided the opportunity to discover truths and illuminate unknowns. I had been unemployed and living off personal savings for six months with dribble income. How long could I continue my lost wanderings? I was saved by Crusader and Tom Richman in particular. They invited me back for some more consulting. What a relief, some solid income again. I could never earn this sort of money with chair massages, acupuncture, and herbal sales and the rocks don't have pain or bleed.

As a geologist, you are at the extremes of the economy. If the economy is doing well, you are doing well, and the reverse applies. Exploration is a risky business with no guarantee of success, and in bad times, risk capital dries up. I was to have forty-six years in the game and was fully employed, apart from the six months in the acupuncture clinic. I had survived by being fleet footed and being prepared to move to chase the work. It was a career of extreme uncertainty, so I kept all our houses at sales pitch in case a quick move was required, and I was forever thinking of alternative employment.

Back in the game and fully focussed, I blossomed. Unlike many other pursuits (sport and chess players come to mind), maturity comes late for a geologist. Experience really does matter. Experience allows for the discernment to understand what is important and what to concentrate on. After my second stint at consulting with Crusader, I took a position with Santos as a development geologist. I had eight invaluable years with them. I found I was working with younger computer savvy people, and I was afforded the opportunity as an older person to receive generous training. This put me in a strong and somewhat unique position as I had the dual edged sword of an extraordinary knowledge of their theatre of operations, the Cooper-Eromanga basin, and I was armed with a digital data base and the computer skills with which to sift and explore for hydrocarbons. I had grown up with this basin. By the time I retired I had been involved for thirty-six years in the exploration and development of oil and gas within the basin.

At Santos, I had the opportunity to fully develop my 'play' concepts as to where best to explore for hydrocarbons. I had a stronger affinity to oil than gas, and I found myself in the favoured position as the only geologist involved in a review of the Santos oil assets in the Queensland sector of the basin. I reviewed all the known oil fields. I was tripping over myself with ideas and possibilities. When the inevitable squeeze arrived, and the only option was a move to Adelaide, I chose the redundancy package and went consulting again. I picked up some varied and amazingly productive work. For a three-year period, I led Victoria Petroleum's exploration in the Cooper Basin, working from my home office while reporting to their Perth office. This was an exciting period in my career, and I was on the well site and called the test resulting in the discovery of Vicpet's first commercial oil field with the drilling of Mirage-1. It was a three-hundred and seventy-two barrels per day oil flow from the Murta Formation. Vicpet had been in the oil game twenty-one years and this was their first discovery and their coming of age. Their managing director and founder, John Kopcheff, had been deprecatingly dubbed 'Dry Hole John' in the oil patch. I was involved with four other discoveries with them, Ventura, Growler, Wirraway, and Snatcher. John was a generous and gregarious character that jokingly said he had bought and sold his Perth house three or four times throughout the ups and downs of the industry with fundraising requirements. He generously provided key people with mementos of discoveries if he considered you had played a part in them. They consisted of a sealed tube of oil in the shape of a droplet encased within a clear epoxy cube. I have five of these that I consider part of my career monuments.

****

With my deep understanding of the basin and well developed 'play' concepts, I applied for vacant and government gazetted acreage in my own private company, financing the applications with consulting income. It takes major capital to conduct oil exploration, capital I did not have, so I became a promoter of acreage. I had an eye for potential, and developed technical arguments, or 'play' concepts, that I then marketed to attract cashed-up joint venture partners. I knew the main players in the industry, and I attended the annual APPEA meetings. I had plenty of mentors that I had observed in the industry over the years, chief of which was Neil Gantry who had won me the Australian Hydrocarbon General Manager position so many years ago. I struck deals culminating in the outright sale of my company.

I had been told I could be Prime Minister one day all my life. I was living off the potential of becoming, but it was always just around the corner, just out of reach. Finally, I had delivered. I had swum with sharks, dined with snakes, and somehow survived. I am forever grateful. I consider I have been very lucky; the Gods have shone on me. Yes, I showed enterprise and I worked hard, but you need things to break your way to make it. I was lucky enough to ride the resources boom for forty-six years.

69

OH, I PLAY SECOND TROMBONE

Irevisited **my ambition to** play the trombone in my early fifties. I made an innocuous, tentative enquiry and rang the Sunnybank Brass Band Secretary,

'Oh hello, um, I sort of play the trombone. Are you looking for any trombonists?'

The secretary replied, 'Can you read treble clef?'

'Yes, that's what I read.' At this stage in my development, this was a mysterious question to ask so I added, 'I only have a small-bore trombone.' It wasn't until much later that I would understand that the trombone is a 'C' pitched instrument with music written on the bass clef, but it can be played as a 'B flat' transposing instrument with music written on the treble clef. In brass bands the first and second tenor trombone parts are written on treble clef. The bass trombone is written on bass clef. Surprisingly, in a brass band it is the only instrument with music written on the bass clef, even tuba music is written on treble clef! In concert bands, every trombone part is written on the bass clef. Good trombonists are required to read not only bass and treble clef music but also alto and tenor clefs, and they must know the slide positions for each note on each clef.

'Well, come along next Monday night and have a blow with the Number two band then, Dennis. We are always looking for new players,' the secretary said.

When I arrived at the band hall on the following Monday night, proudly unfolding my trombone, the secretary had one look at the battered instrument and produced a band instrument for me saying, 'Here, try this. It should make quite a difference to your playing.'

And so I entered the inner sanctum of brass band music fulfilling my desire as a six-year old. I found that there was so much to learn. Watch the conductor, get your phrasing right, don't play as a loner; you are part of a band now. Watch the breath marks… that's where they want you to breathe. To give colour to the music, the conductor moves the tempo around. Don't just get the notes right, you can play them soft, loud, decrescendos, crescendos with sforzando entries. Also watch for the repeat signs: the del capo, the del signo, and coda signs. The No 2 band was a youth band with average age of about sixteen. With greying hair and my regrown moustache, I was unique to this band.

'Listen Dennis, given your experience we'll put you on second trombone,' the conductor said.

'Fine,' I responded. I was simply happy to have the opportunity. I had to bite my lip many a time. I had to learn humility because when you made an error there would be quite a public humiliation. These conductors really know their stuff and always strive for perfection. No playing the piece from top to bottom if something was wrong. They bring the whole band to a stop and correct 'little' and 'not so little' errors then and there.

'You don't swing the hymns, Dennis,' the conductor would bellow.

My brain would be saying, 'Mores the pity, you might be able to make something of them if you did,' but of course these words were never aired.

Coming from a love of jazz, I had developed the bad habit of tapping my foot to the beat of the music. This is a definite 'no-no' in band and orchestral music as it is a major distraction to the conductor and all other players. 'Dennis! I am going to nail that bloody foot of yours to the floor if you move it again!' the conductor repeated for the umpteenth time. It was taking a long time to correct ingrained errors.

You needed skin as thick as a rhinoceros. I had been my own man throughout my career but was now being asked to accept orders from autocratic, demonising conductors. It wasn't easy, but I stuck with it because of my deep love of music.

'Dennis, you're playing that triplet as a semi-quaver. Can you double tongue and triple tongue?' the conductor asked.

What the hell is he talking about? If it's sexual I should know about it by now. This is not a conversation to have in front of the younger people in the band, I was thinking.

'Ah... No,' I responded

'It's called articulation, Dennis. Say after me *'da ga da ga da ga,'* that's double tonguing. Now say *'da da ga, da da ga, da da ga,'* that's triple tonguing. Make sure you can do it by next week.'

'Thanks,' I responded. It sounded like gaga land stuff to me. I was on a fast, steep learning curve.

Then the conductor asked, 'We are a marching band you know. Are you available for the Anzac Day parade?'

'Well, yeah, but I haven't marched before,' I said.

'No problem, it's quite easy. We've got three weeks to Anzac Day and we are scheduling marching practice for the next two Sunday afternoons,' the conductor replied.

I had absolutely no experience in marching. I had not belonged to any military cadet units during my school years. Most brass bands set up with the trombones in the front rank to allow enough room to accommodate their slides. I was still mastering my trombone and now they wanted me to play and march while keeping in line with equal stride lengths with all other band members? And they put me in the front row? Always one to rise to the occasion, I gave it my best shot.

The day arrived, and the band was assembled in George St amongst the diggers for the big parade. Sunnybank took off and capably handled 'On The Road To Gundagai' as we took a right-wheel turn into Adelaide St and approached the main officials' podium within which were the Queensland Governor, the Lord Mayor of Brisbane, and other dignitaries. As instructed, the band had snapped their heads to the left in front of the dignitaries' podium but alas, on returning eyes forward my slide left the trombone. I had forgotten to fasten the little safety clip. As I had played so much football in my youth I managed to gather the slide as it bounced on the road surface in a perfect half volley collect. The drum major, leading the band in front of me, saw the incident and immediately brought the whole band to a halt. With an ever so slight turn of his head and pretending to still look forward, for effect you understand, his neck swelled to overflow his collar and he somehow screwed his mouth around even further and yelled 'Fix it!' One of his now red eyes could be partly seen by me beneath his very military looking little peaked hat. I understood he wasn't exactly happy.

Good command and initiative by the drum major, perhaps, but it was easier said than done. It seemed to me that the eyes of the governor, the lord mayor, and ten thousand spectators were all looking at me. I was awash with sweat running down my legs, at least I hoped it was only sweat, and I was uncontrollably shaking with two pieces of trombone in separate hands trying to get the outer slide onto the inner 'forks' of the slide. Somehow despite the shakes and anxiety the trombone was fixed, and the band completed the march.

At the end of the march, the president of the band who was playing cornet several rows back and was unaware of the drama at the front of the band asked, 'How was that, Dennis? First march, eh?' as he slapped me on the shoulder.

'Great, good fun,' I managed to reply.

'Glad you enjoyed it because we are going to do it again. They are short of bands this year, and we have been asked to go a second time,' he continued.

On the second march through, the band had just completed *'Waltzing Matilda'* as we approached the officials' podium. I had my slide under control and now it was time for the head snap left. I concentrated hard, 'I'll do a super job on this,' I thought. In the next instance I was being admonished from the band member behind saying, 'Dennis, get over. You are way out of line.' I snapped my head forward. *Bloody hell! How has this happened? I've nearly pushed two rows of the band into the gutter in front of the governor,* I thought. The governor in turn was thinking, *How the hell did we manage to win the war?*

There was a lesson to be learnt here. If you look left, you veer left. When snapping head left no need to go to the extreme. Disengage the eyes so that one eye looks left, the other straight ahead. It takes a while to readjust focus on the music held in the lyre inches away after this of course. Nobody passes this sort of key information on. You discover it the hard way.

After a year in the number two band, the organisation took pity on me and I was promoted to the number one band so that I might socialise with the older members. I won awards like '*The Most Improved Player*' and '*The Best Attendance*,' which was very touching but maybe they were playing with my mind a bit.

Some fourteen years on I decided to leave Sunnybank and joined 'Ye Olde Brass Band,' which was composed of retirees. It was a non-competing and non-marching band.

At the first rehearsal I was asked, 'And what do you play, Dennis. First or second?'

'Oh, I play second trombone.'

When I approach the pearly gates I'll immediately inform St Peter, 'I play second trombone.'

It will come as no surprise to me when St Peter replies, 'We know, Dennis. We've been watching!'

EPILOGUE

"The greatest human tragedy is to give up the search"
John Eldredge

EPILOGUE

A geologist's monuments are less tangible than an architect's. My brother, Brian, was a supervising architect on Australia's new parliament house that opened in 1988. He redesigned many overseas embassies. He can look back on his monuments, physically touch them, and gain a tremendous satisfaction of achievement. A geologist's career may be measured on the discoveries to which they are associated. Four achievements stand out in my career which I regard as my monuments.

The first was in 1979 as Beach Petroleum's well site geologist on the discovery well North Paaratte-1; their first commercial hydrocarbons after eighteen years in the game. The field and subsequent adjacent discoveries were developed to supply Warrnambool with enough gas for over twenty years.

Second was being involved with Crusader's triumph over Santos in the legal battle over the 1/1/87 Review and Adjustment, and standing up to the leading petrophysicists of the day in Australia at that time.

My third monument was in 2004, calling the test which resulted in oil to surface for Victoria Petroleum N.L. on Mirage-1. This was their first commercial oil field after twenty-one years of exploration. I subsequently participated in another four oil field discoveries.

My most important monuments, however, are our three loving daughters and three grandchildren. My wish is that they have long, happy and satisfying lives. As I look back on my life I ask what does it all mean? What to conclude?

I am now retired and have the luxury of this more contemplative state. I would say tell some good stories. The fun is in the joint experiences with family and friends and the telling of some good yarns. Honour, remember, and respect with gratitude all the sacrifices that have been made by our forebears as we ride on their shoulders. We owe it to them to do our very best in life, and in that we dutifully honour ourselves.

Mistakes will inevitably be made but do not be despondent. Learn from them, pick yourself up, dust yourself off, and start all over again. A new day is breaking with a new opportunity, seize it. Have faith and believe in yourself. You have the ingredients within to succeed at whatever you want to take on.

Give life a go and take some risks would be my other recommendation to the Harrison clan of the future. Don't die wondering. One of my great joys is playing the card game '500.' It is a trick taking game played with four players playing in pairs that involves team work. It provides lessons in risk taking that tells us so much about ourselves and our opponents. There are no riskless victories. The in-life variant of the populist health fad 'no pain, no gain' is 'no risk, no gain.' A person's approach to risk is revealed in how they play the game of '500.' I played my hand by taking on risk. In the end, there is no alternative. So, with courage, trust, and faith, play your best hand.

Courage comes in so many forms. It takes courage to live and to survive. I have witnessed so many loved ones display enormous courage. Kathy, my mother Hazel, even if I didn't understand that until later in life, and my father Milton. I am a witness to survival. It is somewhat of a miracle that I escaped death several times. I consider I was lucky to have had some fantastic male mentors to guide me along the way, principal of which were Dad, Uncle Ted, Uncle Ron, Dave, Mr Will, and Robbie, but there were many more. These men made me, but countless others have brought me to today and made me who I am now. It is with that understanding that I am in reverent gratitude.

I have been blessed to spend my life with a beautiful and courageous woman, my wife Kathy. We have been a great team, have lived a full life, and endured so much together. We stick like glue and support each other through thick and thin. She knew better than me, as did Michelle Frydenberg, that I would make a very poor politician. It took me a lot longer to understand what her intuition had told her.

Dad, I never made prime minister, but I gave it a go. My wish is that my three grandchildren digest this book, and that it assists them in their approach to life. I say to each of them, 'Kids, you could be prime minister one day.' Grandma and Granddad are in your corner.

"We shall not cease from exploration
And the end of all our exploring
Will be to arrive where we started
And know the place for the first time"

T.S. Eliot

ACKNOWLEDGEMENTS

So many people to thank. This has been a six-year project.

I wish to thank my fellow writers from the Wynnum Creative Writers: Val Gaad, Brenda Campbell, Paula Rees, Judith Ryan, June Beavan, and John Nolan (deceased) for all their critiques in my early efforts. Early editorial advice was received from Pam Collins.

When I ran into deep water, my Boadicea in Pat Noad steered me to shore. Pat, thank you for your encouragement, guidance, wise counsel, and friendship. I would never have made it without you. More importantly, Pat provided an early structural edit.

Then I was fortunate to discover my Richard the Lionheart, Paul Mulligan, who has guided me through so much detail of the publication process. For a new chum, the process is complex, and I have been saved from considerable land mines.

I am also very appreciative of the advice provided by my friend Peter Havord. He has assisted my dwindling spirits with humour at the right time to keep me going forward on the hazardous journey to publication. His constructive feedback has greatly improved the final document.

An accolade to Garry Lock of Simplify Technology, who keeps my computer humming and repairs other IT problems beyond my comprehension.

A thank you to my brother, Brian, who has always provided insight and assisted in numerous discussions on family.

To all the members of my family, thank you for your love and patience in this exercise. I hope to resume normal duties forthwith.

ABOUT THE AUTHOR

I am a writer of short stories and poetry. Under different pennames I have a number of published articles in the Seniors magazine "Your Time" and local newspapers. I live in Brisbane, Australia, with my wife Kathy. Married for over fifty years we have three children and three grandchildren.

Five years ago Kathy and I decided to downgrade to an independent seniors living village called "The Village" at Coorparoo. Best decision we ever made. It is very much the beginning of a new life for us. We are both into keeping fit participating in Pilates, Yoga, Gym work and dancing. I teach Tai Chi and am active in the Variety group and choir. We enjoy travel and are platinum members of our Australian Rules Football team, the Brisbane Lions.

After a successful career as a petroleum exploration geologist I am now pursuing my suppressed love of writing. *"You Could Be Prime Minister One Day Son – Memoir Of A Baby-Boomer"*, is my first full length book.

Thank you for reading my book. If you enjoyed it, won't you please take a moment to leave me a review at your favourite retailer?
Dennis Harrison
Brisbane, 2018

Made in the USA
Middletown, DE
30 June 2018